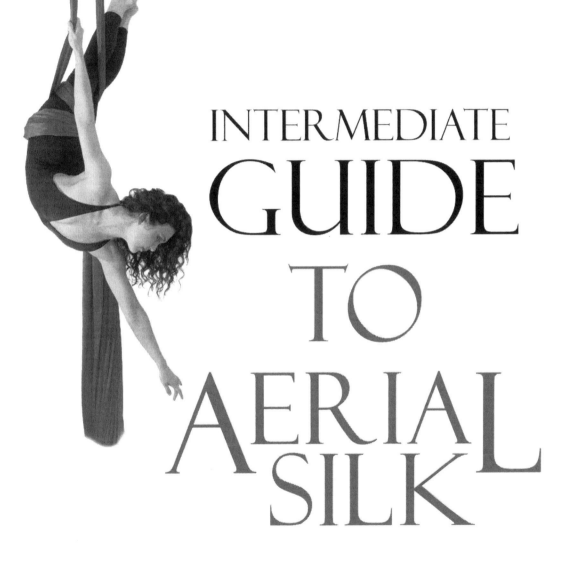

INTERMEDIATE GUIDE TO AERIAL SILK

—JILL FRANKLIN—
Owner of Aerial Physique

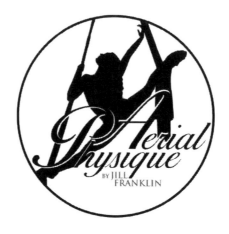

Intermediate Guide to Aerial Silk

Copyright © 2015 by Jill Franklin

Printed in the United States of America

ISBN: 978-0-692-54846-2

Please Note:
This book has been written and published strictly for informational purposes, and in no way should it be used as a substitute for live instruction with a professional.

USE THIS BOOK AT YOUR OWN RISK

DEDICATION

I dedicate this book to my husband, true love really does make it all possible!
A special THANK YOU to all of you who supported by first book,
you are the reason for this second book!

Table of Contents

PREFACE

Dear Aerialist,

My romance with aerial began many years ago when I saw my first Cirque du Soleil show at the age of fourteen. I was mesmerized by the beauty, grace and strength the performers displayed. At the time I assumed one would have to grow up in a circus school, spending hours a day training away to achieve such skill. I only had a background in ballet and did not possess the skill set to duplicate what I had admired on stage. Little did I know then, that years later I would be performing similar aerial feats in front of thousands of people in beautiful theaters throughout the world.

When I first began aerial in my early 20s in New York City, I was terrible. I lacked the upper body strength and coordination. With consistent practice, patience and belief in myself, I eventually overcame my limits with strength and achieved my skill on a professional level.

I have a passion for helping others and feel the same romance that I do with aerial. My background in ballet, classical Pilates and yoga all encompass my Aerial Physique technique. The key to any worthwhile fitness endeavor is strength, flexibility and cardiovascular activity. Aerial work has it all! The best part about it, it's incredibly rewarding and fun!

The book I have designed is for the intermediate level aerialist who would like to deepen their understanding of aerial silk work. It is not intended as the sole learning avenue. It is best to always practice with a qualified instructor. I wish for you to be patient, consistent and kind to yourself while learning. Enjoy, be safe and most of all have fun!

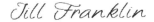

i

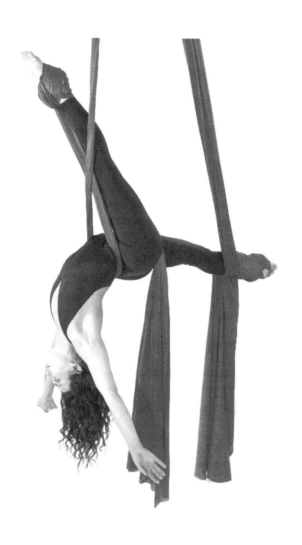

INTRODUCTION

What is aerial silk? Aerial silk (aka: fabric, tissu) is a beautiful art form and evolving fitness craze. Practitioners of this strength building craft climb, invert and wrap their bodies into and out of various positions stemming from gymnastics and ballet. It can also be referred to as aerial acrobatics, aerial dance or aerial fitness.

Aerial acrobatics has been performed in the circus for thousands of years. The modern world began to take note of this stunning art form in 1998 when Cirque du Soleil's show *Quidam* displayed an aerial silk contortion act on red fabric. Since then, many circus schools, dance companies and most recently fitness studios and gyms have been offering classes in aerial silk.

This book introduces you to the intermediate level skills, positions and movements involved in aerial silk work. There are countless variations within intermediate level silk work. The ones I have chosen for this guide are some of my personal favorites and the thousands of students I've instructed over the years agree. I have come across many different names for the feats in this book, you may have learned them by another name. Throughout this guide you will see AKA (also known as) feel free to write in the name of the trick or movement which is most familiar to you.

The ascent into artistry demonstrated within, are building blocks for more advanced variations and combinations. Take your time and learn thoroughly. ALWAYS practice clean technique and proper form. It is much more impressive to do the feats smooth and controlled, versus throwing yourself into things too soon and potentially getting injured or tangled in the fabric!

Keep an eye out for upcoming DVDs and books from Aerial Physique. Join the Aerial Physique video tutorial membership site and gain access to hundreds of tutorial videos. Visit www.aerialphysique.com to sign up. Subscribe to the Aerial Physique YouTube Channel for instructional videos by Jill Franklin.

AERIAL FOUNDATION

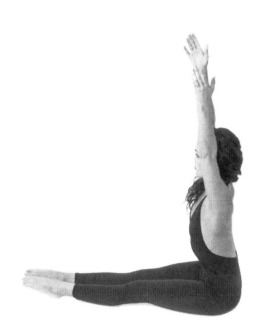

Aerial Movement Principles

1. Safety: Aerial is a potentially dangerous activity that can cause injury or even death. Make sure that you are suspended on an apparatus that has been installed by a licensed rigger and always practice with a professional instructor. Know you limits. If you find you are tired stop and rest. It is best to be safe then push yourself too far.

2. Concentration: The key element to connecting your mind and body is concentration. Aerial work is both a physical and mental practice. It is extremely important to be present in your mind while learning and executing movements. You will progress much more rapidly while having a safer approach to the task at hand.

3. Precision: Practice makes perfect. Proper form is essential to ensure you achieve the beautiful lines of the positions while preventing injury.

4. Control: In aerial work, control of your entire body is the name of the game. No sloppy or haphazard movements are allowed.

5. Centering: By paying attention to the muscles of the core (abdominals, lower back, hips and glutes) you will help all of your bodies' muscles function and develop more efficiently.

6. Breathing: Controlling your breath with deep exhalations as you perform aerial movements helps activate your muscles and keep you focused. When you are upside down it is very easy to forget to breath!

7. Balance: A truly balanced body has an equal amount of strength and flexibility. Muscles should be supple, mobile, yet strong. Flexibility and range of motion are important components in aerial work.

8. Flow: In time aerial work becomes continuous flowing movement. An "aerial dance". Each movement, position and transition should be smooth and graceful. In the beginning movements may feel awkward and jerky, allow yourself plenty of practice and soon you will be flowing with ease!

Aerial Terminology

Aerial: Performed in the air.

Arabesque: A ballet position made by balancing on the supporting leg, while extending the free leg behind with a straight knee.

Attitude: A ballet position made by standing on one leg, while the other leg is lifted and turned out with the knee bent at approximately a 90 degree angle.

Carabiner: A metal loop with a spring-loaded gate used in rigging aerial apparatus.

Crochet: A term used in aerial silk work when wrapping your arms or legs from the outside around the fabric and securing the position using your hand or foot.

Foot Positions: The positioning of the feet is particularly important in aerial. Your feet will be pointed in most cases to finish the line of the positions. For some positions flexed or sickled feet will be an anchor in which you are hanging from.

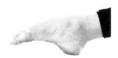

Pointed Foot   **Flexed Foot**   **Sickled Foot**

Pike: A gymnastics term meaning bent forward at the hips.

Pilates: A physical fitness system developed in the early 20th century by Joseph Pilates. He called his method "Contrology" the art of control.

Planche: A gymnastics skill in which the body is held parallel to the ground, giving the illusion of floating. There are many variations of the planche in aerial work.

Pole of the silk: The secure or tight part of the fabric. Usually referring to the piece of fabric above your locked point (foot lock, hip key, ect.). AKA: Live End

Rescue 8: An aerial hardware piece which the fabric is wrapped around.

Rond de jambe: A French ballet term meaning circular movement of the leg.

Rosin: A form of resin derived from pine trees, used to help gripping ability in aerial work. It is available in powered and spray forms.

Silks: A term for the fabric used in aerial work. The fabric type is a strong two way stretch nylon tricot. It comes in an array of colors and stretch depending on the needs of the aerialist.

Splits: A position in which the legs are in line with each other and extended in opposite directions.

Straddle: A position in which the legs are open towards a V shape or wider.

Swivel: A hardware piece used in rigging single point aerial apparatus. It keeps the fabric in rotation and prevents it from getting twisted when in use.

Tail of the silk: The dangling part of the fabric that is below your locked point. AKA: Dead End

Tissu: Translates into "fabric" in French.

The following symbols will be seen throughout the book:

★   **Final Position**

🚫   **Incorrect**

TIPS: The tip box provides helpful tips & more details

AKA: Also known as & fill in what you know the trick as

Your Aerial Muscles

Aerial work utilizes primarily the upper body and abdominals. Pictured below are some of the large muscles that are worked when doing aerial activities. Although in some movements the entire body is engaged, these are the main muscles at work.

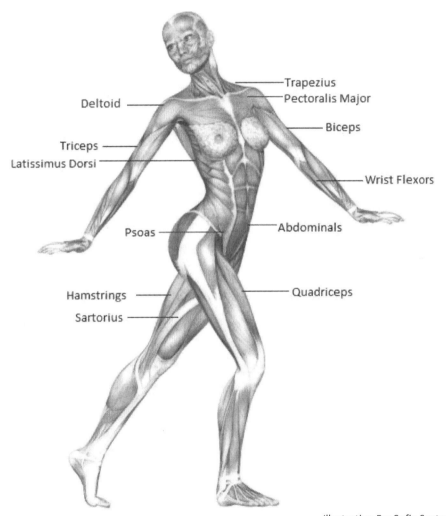

Illustration By: Sofia Santos

Abdominals: There are four muscles that make up the abdominal wall. All are extremely important in aerial work. **Transverse**, the deepest of the four assists in stabilizing the spine and forcing air out of the lungs. The **internal and external obliques** assist in rotating, flexing and side bending movements. Lastly the **rectus,** also known as the "six pack", works to flex (bend) the trunk.

Biceps: The front of the upper arm, it bends and supinates (turns palm upwards) the forearm. It is active during chin ups.

Deltoid: A shoulder muscle that assists in lifting the arm away from the body.

Hamstrings: A group of three muscles in the back of the leg that bend the knee and extend (straighten) the thigh. When flexible, this muscle group makes achieving a pike position is easy.

Latissimi Dorsi: Meaning "Widest Back Muscle" it is your climbing and pull up muscle. Also known as the "lats", your wings in aerial.

Pectoralis Major: Your main chest muscle, at work when doing push-ups.

Psoas: Deep hip flexor muscle that flexes the thigh and turns out the leg.

Quadriceps: The front of your thigh. A group of four muscles that assist in straightening the knee and flexing the thigh.

Sartorius: The inner thigh. It is the longest muscle in the body. Turns out the hips. When flexible achieving a straddle position is easy.

Trapezius: Upper, middle and lower traps work to move the shoulder blades up and down. They also work when holding the arm to the side or overhead.

Triceps: The back of the upper arm, it extends (straightens) the forearm. At work in many aerial feats.

Wrist Flexors: The forearm. Bends wrists towards the body. They are your grip muscles in aerial and are worked tremendously!

PREPARING FOR AERIAL

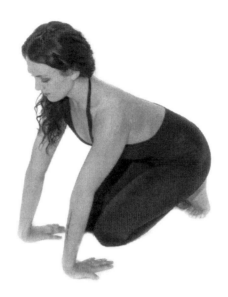

Warming Up

It is highly important to include a proper warm up prior to any aerial activities. An effective warm up heats the body and includes movements in all ranges of motion including flexion (forward bending), extension (back bending), side bending and twisting. A Pilates, ballet or gymnastics based warm up are all great options. You could also do something as simple as jogging in place or jumping jacks followed by the strength building positions and stretches as pictured in the pages to come.

Core strength is crucial in aerial work. The positions to come demonstrate the correct and incorrect alignment during core work or in Pilates terms your "Powerhouse." Proper recruitment of your abdominals, lower back, hips and glutes are all vital when working your core.

Proper Hollow Body Position
Hollow body is a gymnastics term and a fundamental position used in aerial work. Once you progress holding this shape begin to reach your arms up by your ears keeping your neck in neutral alignment.

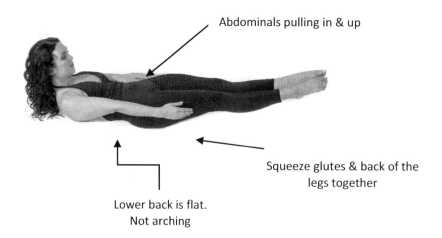

Abdominals pulling in & up

Squeeze glutes & back of the legs together

Lower back is flat.
Not arching

Incorrect Hollow Body Position

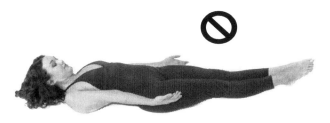

Proper Plank Position

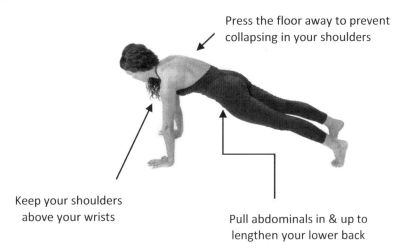

Press the floor away to prevent collapsing in your shoulders

Keep your shoulders above your wrists

Pull abdominals in & up to lengthen your lower back

Incorrect Plank Position

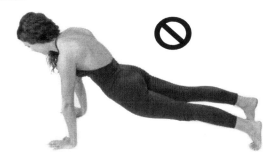

Stretching

Seated Pike

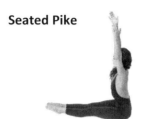 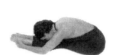

Forearm Stretch

Straddle

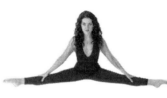 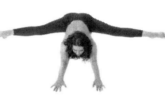

Middle Splits

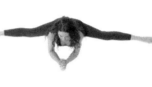

Splits

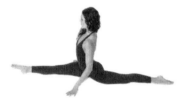 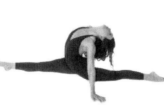

Over Splits

Back Bending

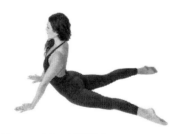 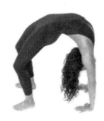 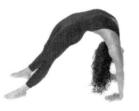

Grip & Arm Options

Proper Grip

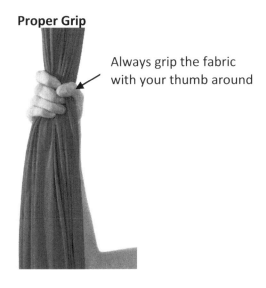

Always grip the fabric with your thumb around

Incorrect Grip

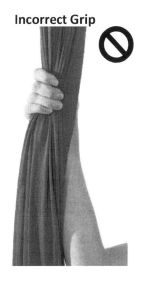

Correct Shoulder Placement

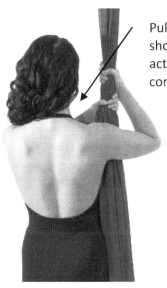

Pulling your shoulders down activates the correct muscles

Incorrect Shoulder Placement

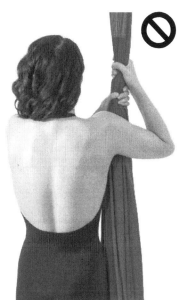

When practicing aerial it is important to always remember these two fundaental components.

Bent Arms vs Straight Arms

Knowing the difference between working with bent arms versus straight arms is extremely important. At times when we are tired or unsure of a move, we end up working somewhere in between these two places. It is crucial that we are clear in what version we are using to properly strengthen our muscles and prevent injury.

Bent Arms

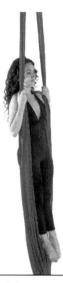

Straight Arms

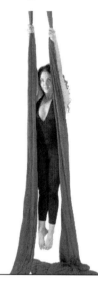

Working with bent arms is the most common position within this book. It is used for most beginner and intermediate level tricks. Bent arms mainly activates the triceps, lats (latissimus dorsi) biceps and grip muscles. When working in this position bring your elbows in towards your hips, pull your shoulders away from your ears, keep your shoulders open (not hunched forward) and maintain a hollow body position.

Working with straight arms is typically a more advanced way of working with the exception of the classic climb. Straight arms mainly activates the lats (latissimus dorsi), shoulder and grip muscles. When working in this position keep space around your neck by gently pulling your shoulders away from your ears and maintain a hollow body position.

Grip Options Between the Fabrics

1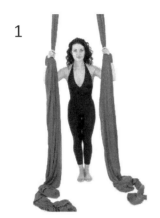

2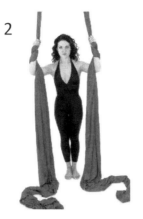

3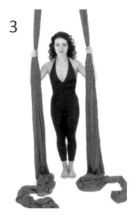

Most Grip Support
Locked Wrist Keys

Hug the fabric, flip it
over your wrist, turn
your hand in towards
the fabric and grab
creating a lock.

Some Grip Support
Circle Twice-Outside In

Hug the fabric, circle
your wrists upwards
around it twice.

No Grip Support
Holding

Simply grip the fabric.

**Choose one of the grip support choices above, for the
positions shown in the coming pages. As your grip gets
stronger, eventually all of the coming shapes can be
performed in the air by simply gripping the fabric.**

Climbing Grip Option - Split Finger Climb

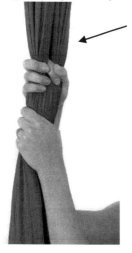

Place your index finger in between the fabrics

The split finger grip can be used when your first trick in the air is with the fabrics open (splits, candy cane, inverting in between fabrics etc.). It takes away the worry of fussing with the fabrics when trying to find the center. When using this in a climb, keep your same hand on the top.

Flamenco Grip

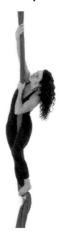

From a right side climb, reach your right arm up and around the fabric with your thumb facing up. Internally rotate your shoulder so you have space to grab the fabric. For some, this feels impossible for your wrist, internally rotating your shoulder will help!

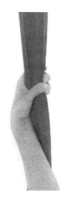

The flamenco grip is used as a quick way to get into positions such as (arabesque) and for a (S-Wrap) entry.
Warm up your wrists and shoulders before attempting this.

WARM UP SHAPES

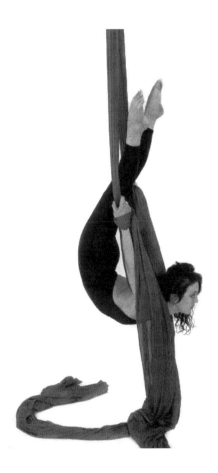

Please see more basic warm up shapes in *Beginners Guide to Aerial Silk*

Bird's Nest

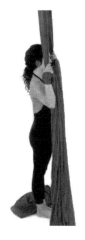

1

Choose your grip option. Begin in between the fabrics.

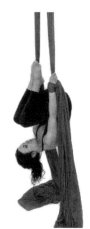

2

Invert into a tuck.

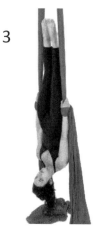

3

Straighten your legs up into a candlestick.

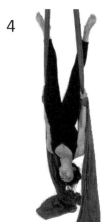

4

Open your legs and press your shins against the back of the fabric.

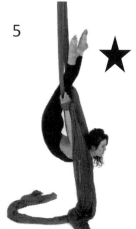

5 ★

Press your hips forward and arch your upper back.

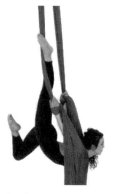

Single Leg Option:
Sickle one foot around the fabric and bend your opposite knee towards your chest.

TIPS
*Press your shins against the fabric versus hooking your feet, it creates a much nicer line
*A sickled foot on the single leg variation is necessary to secure the position
* It is easy to get confused which side of the fabric to put your legs, look up so you see where you are placing them when learning   AKA: _____

Inverted Splits

1

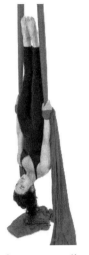

Begin from a candlestick
position.

2

★

Open your legs into a split keeping
your hips square and forearms
pressing into your sides. Once
your legs are in position arch your
upper back.

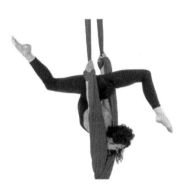

Stag Option:
Bend your knees creating a
stag position.

```
TIPS
*You have to have an over-split on the floor to achieve a flat
inverted split in the air
*Keep your hips square in between the fabrics
*Pressing your arms into your sides helps to secure the position
*The double stag option creates a nice line and works well if you don't
have a flat inverted split
*Practice this on both sides
AKA: _____
```

Angel

1

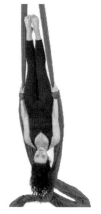

Begin from a
candlestick
position.

2

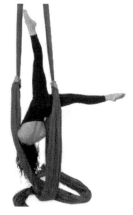

Keep your right leg in the
center and bring your left
leg forward creating an
upside down arabesque.

3 ★

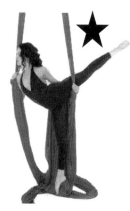

Drop your right
leg down and pull
up with your
right arm.

4

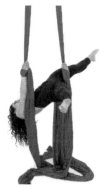

To come out, drop
your shoulders back
the way you came.

5

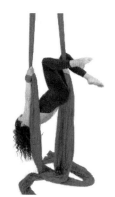

Tuck your right
knee in followed by
your left.

6

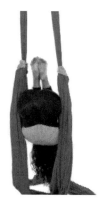

End in a tuck.
Repeat on your
other side.

TIPS

*This requires pull up strength and understanding of an arabesque position

*Think of doing a pull up with your right arm in step 3, it will help you to get your torso up

*Keep your left hand next to your inner thigh, it is common to let it slide down to the knee

AKA: Eagle _____

CLIMBING

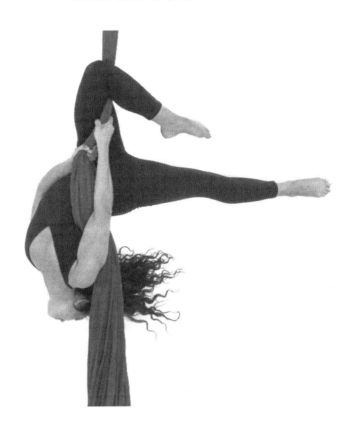

Classic Climb - L Roll Up

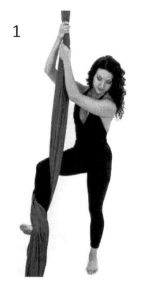

1

Wrap your right leg around the fabric from the outside in.

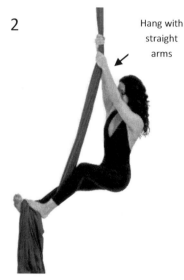

2

Hang with straight arms

Step your left foot on top of your right using the ball of your foot creating a L shape.

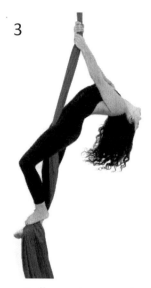

3

Roll your torso up by pressing your hips forward and arching your upper back.

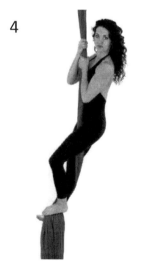

4

Stand up. Reach your arms up and repeat.

TIPS

*Press your feet forward when stepping up to climb versus down

*Allow your legs to help you out versus depending solely on your arms

*Lifting your knees up high into your chest between each climb will help you gain height versus pulling up with your arms

*Reach your arms up high in between each climb, it is easier to roll up if your arms are high

*Rolling upward provides a more artistic look versus a standard climb

*When rolling up lead with your hips allowing your head to be the last to lift

AKA:_____

Classic Climb Descent

Version #1 Port de bras Decent

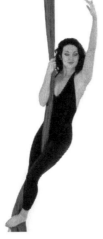

1

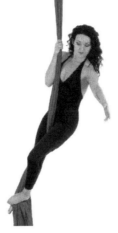

2

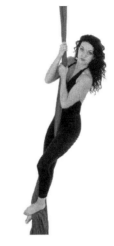

3

Begin with your hands in front of your chest. Release your top hand and reach your arm up.

Circle your arm out to the side.

Grab underneath your other hand. Repeat on the opposite side.

Version #2 Hand over Hand Decent

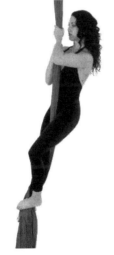

1

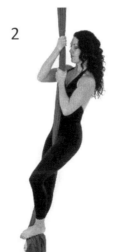

2

Walk your hands down the fabric while lightening the tension between your feet.

TIPS
*To avoid getting a fabric burn don't slide your hands down the fabric, instead, move them one at a time
*Eventually there are several ways to descend down the fabric, these two are the most basic
*Port de bras means "carriage of the arms" in ballet terminology

AKA:_____

Straddle Descent

1
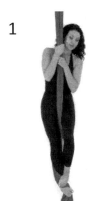

Begin from a classic climb with your hands in front of your chest.

2 3
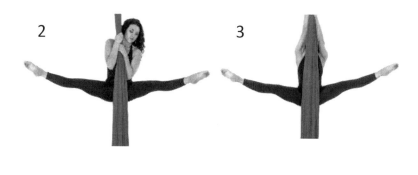

Release your feet from the fabric and open your legs into a straddle.

Slowly lower down until your arms are straight keeping your legs in a straddle.

4
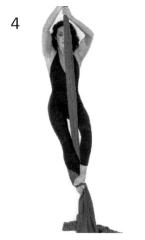

Re-wrap your feet for the classic climb. Repeat.

TIPS
*Turn your legs out from your hips and slightly tuck your pelvis under in your straddle to recruit your lower abs
*Lowering down slowly is great for strengthening your upper body, it is referred to as a "negative pull up"
*Watch that your shoulders don't hunch by your ears when taking your feet off the fabric, instead slide your shoulder blades down your back and lengthen your neck
*Do your best to keep your legs lifting in your straddle during steps 2-3
* Repeat on your other side with your opposite hand on top
AKA:_____

Arch Descent

1
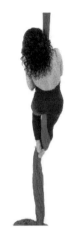

Begin from a classic climb with hands in front of your chest.

2
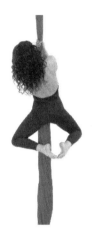

Take your feet off the fabric in a diamond shape behind you.

3
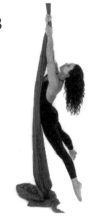

Slowly lower down until your arms are straight, lengthen your legs behind you and lift your chest up.

4
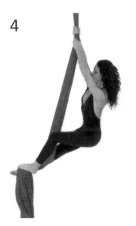

Re-wrap your feet for the classic climb. Repeat.

TIPS
*Lowering down slowly is great for strengthening your upper body, it is referred to as a "negative pull up"
*Press your hips forward and slightly lift your chest up, (see step 3) to create a nice line in the body
*This can be used as a conditioning climb or in choreography
*Repeat on your other side with your opposite hand on top
AKA:_____

Glissade Descent

1

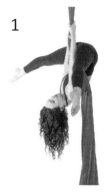

Invert in a straddle with the fabric on your right side.

2

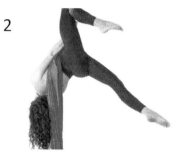

Hook your right knee above your hands while turning your left leg behind you.

3

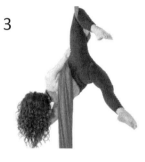

Release your left hand and reach for the tail of the fabric with a "back stroke" motion.

4

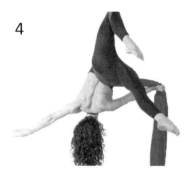

Grab the tail of the fabric with your left hand, palm up and open your arm to the side creating a "shelf" for your lower back. Once your left hand is secure release your right hand.

5

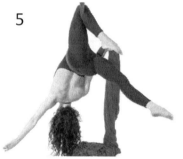

Slightly loosen the grip in your left hand allowing yourself to slide. Once you are near the ground hold tightly and bring your left arm next to your body.

6

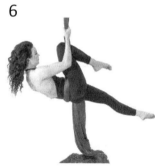

To come out, climb above your right knee or exit into a back balance, see page 85.

6

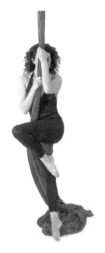

Press your hips forward
creating a "thigh hitch"
around your right thigh.

7

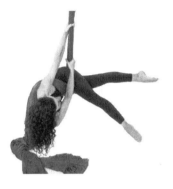

Drop your torso to the
right and swim the tail
behind your back with
your left arm.

TIPS
*Make sure your lower back is covered when doing this, steps 4-5 can
create a fabric burn
*Be sure that your palm faces up during steps 4-5
*Square your hips to face upwards
*You can also exit step 5 into a back balance (see page 85)
*Keep your arm straight to the side maintaining the shelf on your lower
Back
*The term "swim" (see step 7) is a commonly used term among aerialists,
meaning, place the fabric behind your back using a "back stroke" motion
AKA:_____

Climbing In Between the Fabrics

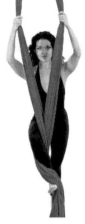

1

Begin with the fabrics open. Wrap your right leg in the classic climb position.

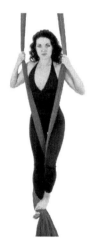

2

Step your left foot on top of your right.

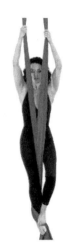

3

Reach your arms up one at a time.

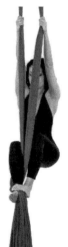

4

Hang with straight arms, lift your knees to your chest and re-wrap your feet.

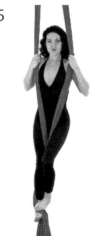

5

Push your feet forward to stand up. Repeat.

TIPS
*This is a great climb to use for tricks that begin in the air between the fabrics
*You can make this more artistic by making a L shape and rolling your body up in the fabric
*Repeat using your opposite foot to climb
*Another variation, pull up in between each climb instead of keeping your arms straight
AKA:_____

Bicycle Climb

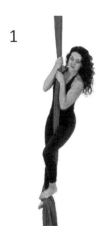

1

Begin from a classic climb on your right.

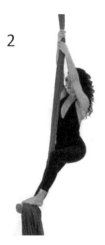

2

Reach your arms up and drop your hips away from the fabric.

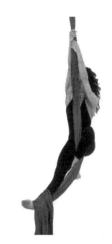

3

Lift your left foot up and crochet it inside the pole of the fabric, place the fabric on the arch of your foot.

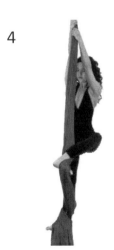

4

Press your left foot forward maintaining a flexed foot and a turned out leg. Keep the tail of the fabric draped over your right foot.

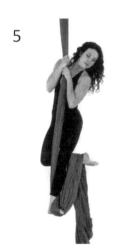

5

Pull up and put weight onto your left foot. Bend your right knee keeping the tail draped over your heel.

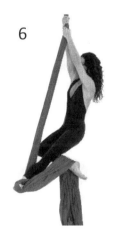

6

Reach your arms up, drop your hips back.

7	8	9
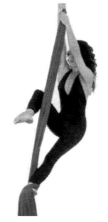	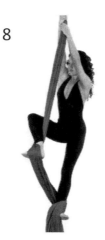	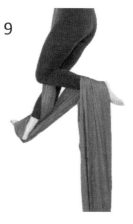
Allow the tail to fall off your right heel.	Crochet your right foot inside, placing the fabric on your arch.	Put weight into your right foot, bringing your left heel towards your tush. Repeat.

TIPS
*This climb is a tricky one! Be clear about every step
*Make sure the fabric is on the arch of your foot when pressing forward in steps 4 & 8, it can easily slide up around your ankle
*In step 5 it is important to keep the tail draped over your back heel and bring your heel towards your tush with your knees together to avoid slipping
*You can use this climb to take a standard single foot lock off
AKA: Ladder Climb _____

Same Side Straddle Inversion Climb

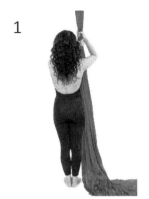

1

Begin with the fabric on your right side.

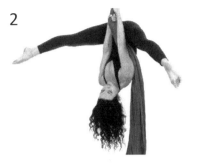

2

Invert in a straddle keeping the tail to the right.

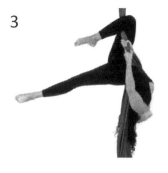

3

Hook your right knee above your hands. Rotate your left leg behind you.

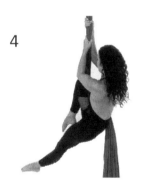

4

Climb above your right knee leading with your right hand.

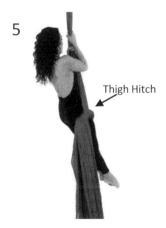

5

Thigh Hitch

Pull up and press your hips forward until you feel the knot slide up high around your right thigh, creating a thigh hitch.

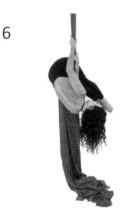

6

Drop your torso to the right pressing your left hip (top hip) into the pole of the fabric. Choose your leg option, see page 31.

7

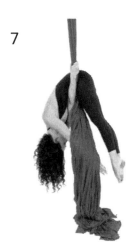

Using the back of your left forearm begin to swim the fabric behind you. Option: Hold the pole of the fabric with your right hand for extra safety.

8

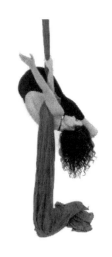

Continue to swim until the fabric is on your back.

9

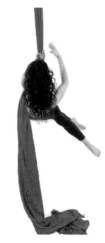

Grab the pole of the fabric with your left hand followed by your right.

10

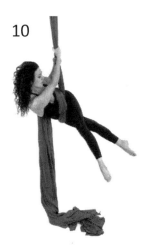

Place your hands close together.

11

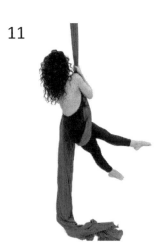

Pull your chest close to the fabric, lower your legs and the fabric will fall off.

12

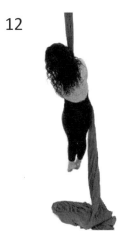

Hang with your arms bent, the tail on your right side. Repeat by inverting.

Leg Options for Thigh Hitch

(during steps 6-10)

Scissor Legs
Most Secure Option

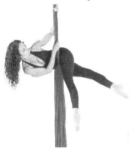

Scissor legs provide the most secure position when swimming the fabric behind your back and for movements such as hip key. The options below are doable but do not provide as much support which may entail sliding down the fabric. Your clothing and the weather (the fabric is affected by the climate) are factors in these position choices.

| Pike | Tuck | Single Leg Cross Over |

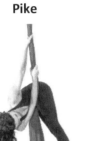 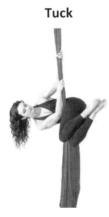 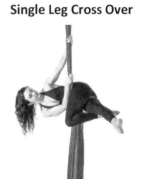

When inverting in a straddle DO NOT invert with the fabric between your legs. Always keep the fabric to the side of your body.

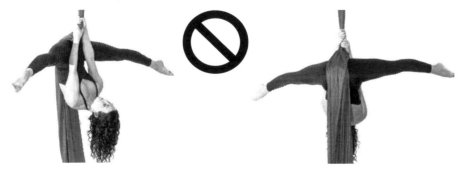

TIPS

*Be sure NOT to hook your knee on top of your hands, this is extremely dangerous, instead hook your knee above your hands

*If it is too challenging to invert with straight legs, then pass your knees through a diamond shape until you build strength

*The fabric will always stay on the same side for this climb, it does not alternate sides in the air, hence the name "same side climb"

*When climbing above your knee, keep your hooked leg in the same place, if you allow it to drop, you will slide

*It is vital to press your hips forward (see step 5) to allow the knot to slide up as high as possible creating a "thigh hitch." If you do not press your hips forward enough you will most likely slide when moving to step 6

*During step 10 place your hands on the fabric at approx. eye level, if you reach them up too high you will have to do a straight arm inversion which is very challenging at the intermediate level

*If you are working on 16-20 foot ceilings you should be able to get to the top in 2-3 climbs

AKA: _____

**"Practice does not make perfect.
Only perfect practice makes perfect."**
Vince Lombardi

Opposite Side Inversion Climb

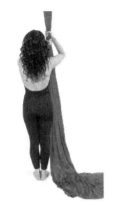

1

Begin with the fabric on your right side.

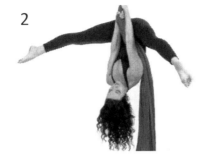

2

Invert to a straddle keeping the fabric to your right.

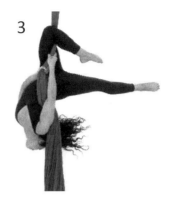

3

Hook your left knee above your hands and rotate your right leg behind you.

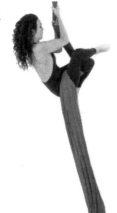

4

Climb above your left knee leading with your left hand. The moment you release your right hand to climb above cross your right leg over your left.

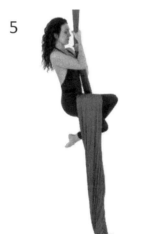

5

Pull up keeping your legs crossed. The tail will be on your right, hold the pole of the fabric towards your left side.

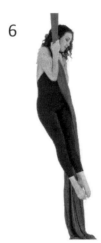

6

Pull your elbows in toward your sides and release the cross of your legs. The fabric will fall off.

6

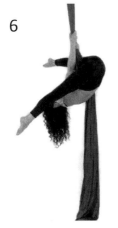

Invert with the tail to your left. Hook your right knee above your hands repeat steps 3-5.

"Obstacles are those frightful things you see when you take your eyes off your goal."

Henry Ford

In Between Fabrics Knee Climb

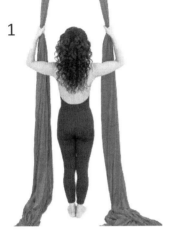

1

Begin standing in between the fabrics.

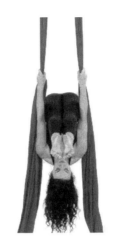

2

Invert between into a pike.

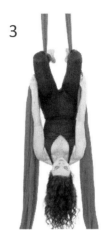

3

Hook both knees above your hands.

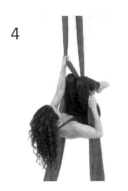

4

Squeeze the fabric in the back of your knees by pressing your heels towards your tush. Reach one hand above your knee.

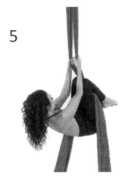

5

Reach the other hand above your knee.

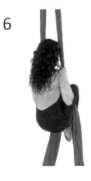

6

Pull up into a tuck position.

7

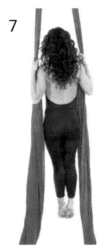

Lengthen your legs beneath you
and the fabric will fall off.

8

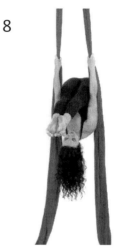

Repeat by inverting into a pike in
between the fabrics.

TIPS
*Don't underestimate the knee squeeze!
*To make it easier you can pass through a tuck before extending your legs in a pike (see step 2)
*In some cases putting rosin on the backs of your knees can help prevent slipping if you find your legging/tights are not cooperating
*You don't have to begin standing in between the fabrics, this can also be done mid-air
AKA: _____

In Between Fabrics Knee Climb - One Side

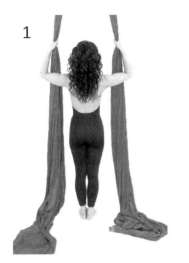

Begin standing in between the fabrics.

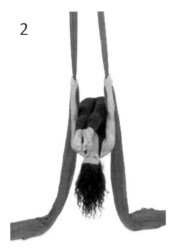

Invert in between the fabrics into a pike position.

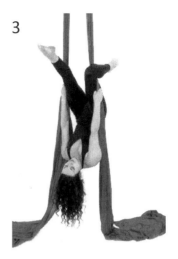

Hook the back of your right knee above your right hand.

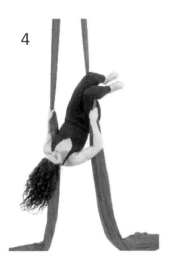

Quickly hook the back of your left knee above your right.

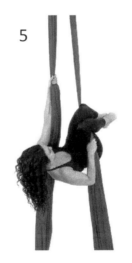

Reach your left hand higher on the left fabric.

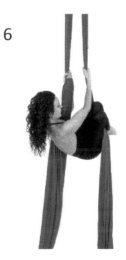

Squeeze the fabric behind your knees and reach your right hand above.

7

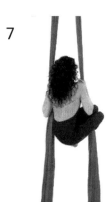

Pull up and bring your
torso in between the
fabrics.

8

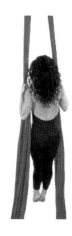

Release your feet
from the fabric and
lengthen your legs.
Repeat.

TIPS
*You can alternate sides while in the air or stay on the same side
*It gives you a much better grip placing one leg on the fabric at a time (steps 3-4)
versus both knees at the same time
*Don't underestimate the knee squeeze!
*To make it easier you can pass through a tuck before extending your legs in a
pike (see step 2)
*In some cases putting rosin on the backs of your knees can help prevent slipping
if your leggings/tights are not cooperating
*You don't have to begin standing in between the fabrics, this can also be done
mid-air
AKA:_____

FOOT LOCK POSITIONS & TRICKS

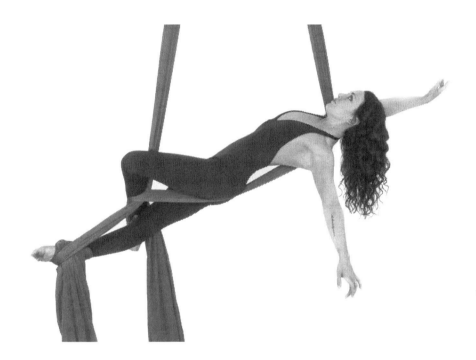

Candy Cane

1

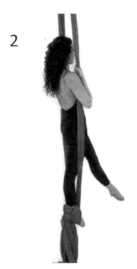

Begin from a single foot lock on the right.

2

Separate the fabrics and bring your hips in between.

3

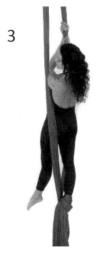

Place both hands on the right side.

4

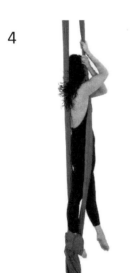

Turn and face the right fabric.

5

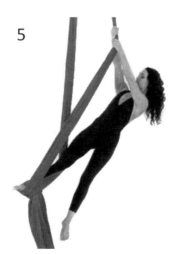

Drop your torso in between the fabrics with your chest facing up. The left fabric will slide to the back of your knee.

6

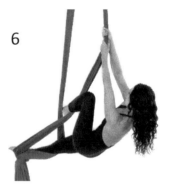

Lift your left leg up and begin to press the fabric on your right side down using the outside of your foot.

7

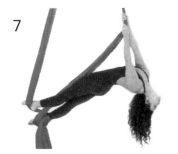

Press the fabric down to
your ankle and arch your
upper back.

8

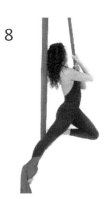

Pull up and roll
to the right to
complete your 1st
leg roll.

9

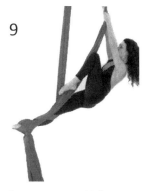

Repeat steps 5-6.

10

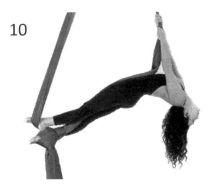

Press the fabric down to your
ankle and arch your upper back.

11

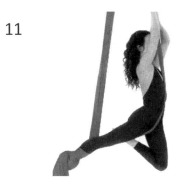

Pull up and roll to the right to
complete your 2nd leg roll.

12

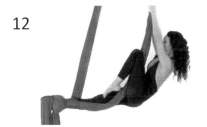

Continue rolling to complete
your 3rd roll. If done correctly
you shouldn't have to press the
fabric down.

13

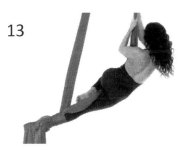

Roll to the right, the fabric should
be around your lower leg, not
around your knee.

14

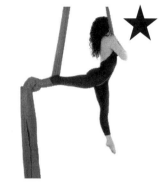

Arrive in the complete
candy cane shape.

15

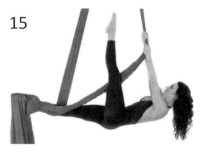

To come out, roll to the left
making a fan kick motion with
your left leg. Pull up between
each roll.

16

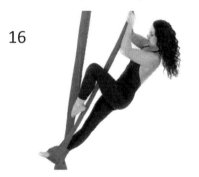

Continue to unroll 3½ times.

17

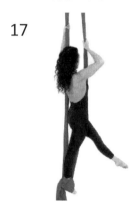

Arrive in between the
fabrics.

18

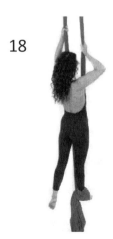

Bring your left leg back out
in between the fabrics.

19

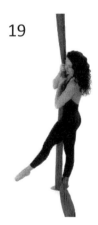

End in a single foot lock.

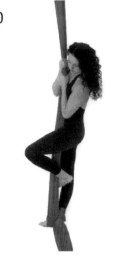

Take your foot lock off using the outside of your left foot.

TIPS

*Use the outside of your foot (versus your arch) to press the fabric down, this allows for a smooth transition

*Make sure your arms are not too low when rolling up, grabbing a bit higher in between each roll can be beneficial

*Keep your leg that is in the foot lock straight the entire time

* The fabric can get stuck on your calf muscle if your lower legs are bare. Wearing long leggings or tights is helpful

*If you feel it is too much to roll up three times then just roll twice

*If it's too difficult to keep your leg fan kicking leg straight when rolling out, then bend your knee to unwind

*When rolling out don't miss the half turn! If you rolled up 3 times unroll 3 ½ if you rolled up to 2 times then 2 ½, not fully unrolling will result in you possibly getting stuck!

AKA: Man on the Moon, Twirly Bird

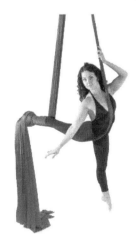

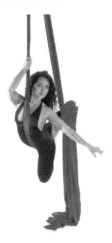

Figure 4

1

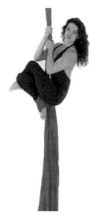

From a single foot
lock in the air squat
down with the fabric
in between your legs.

2

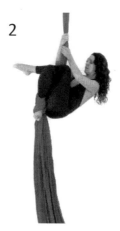

Squeeze your inner
thighs together as
you lean back.

3

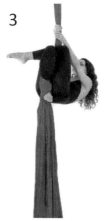

Place the fabric
just below your
right knee.

4

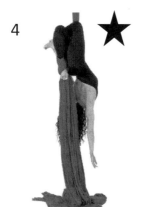

Keep your legs
crossed and
squeezing together
as you lean back.
Option: Hold the top
of your right foot
when leaning back.

5

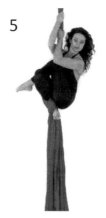

Sit all the way up.

TIPS
*Squeeze your inner
thighs together!
*You can hold your
right ankle with your
right hand to secure
the position
*It takes core
strength to sit back
up, commit to it!
AKA: Ladysit Hang

Lay Back Split

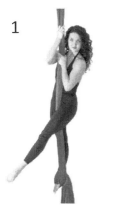

1

Begin from a single foot lock.

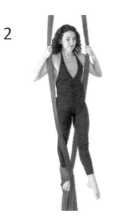

2

Open the fabrics, bring your hips in between and your left leg forward.

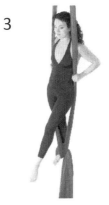

3

Move your hands down next to your waist.

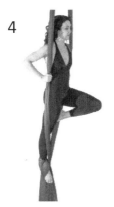

4

Bend your left knee towards your chest.

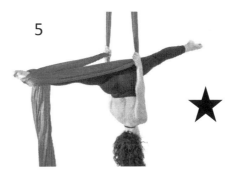

5

Slowly arch backwards, extend your left leg into a split.

6

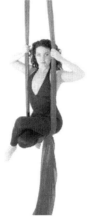

To come out bend your right knee and sit in between the fabrics crossing your left leg over your right.

7

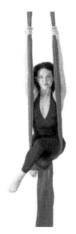

Reach your arms up.

8

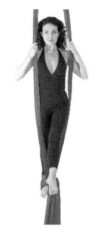

Pull up and stand.

TIPS
*Move slowly in step 5 and stop when your right leg (back leg) is horizontal to the floor, going too quickly or losing the tension on the fabric can result in an accidental 360 flip!
*An over split on the floor Is necessary to achieve a flat inverted split in the air
*Step 6 can also serve as a resting position, additional choreography can be added during this step
AKA: Upside Down Splits _____

Arabesque

Entry #1

1

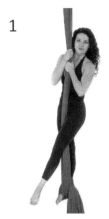

Begin from a single foot lock on the right.

2

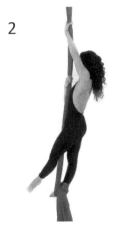

Reach your left arm up using a flamenco grip (see page 14).

3

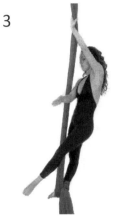

Pass your right arm in the space between you and the fabric.

4

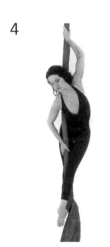

Place your right shoulder in front of the fabric.

5

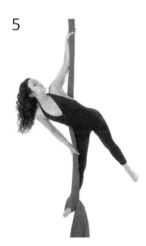

Lean forward until you feel the pole of the fabric on your lower back.

6 ★

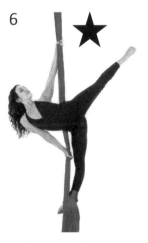

Lift your left leg up behind you into an arabesque.

7

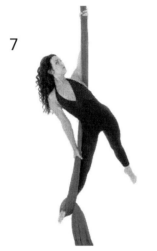

To come out slightly lower your left leg down behind you.

8

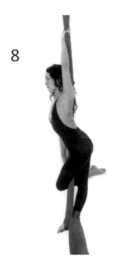

Pass your shoulders back the way you came.

9

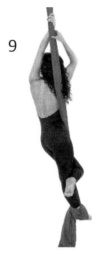

Meet your right hand with your left and turn around the pole of the fabric.

10

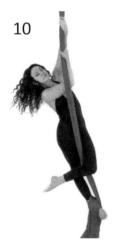

Continue to turn until the fabric is in front of you.

11

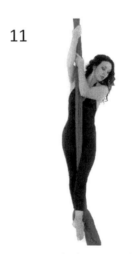

Switch the grip of your right hand followed by your left.

TIPS
*The flamenco grip (see page 14) can be tricky for some, if your wrist does not agree with it try entry #2
*When you arrive in your arabesque (step 6) press your lower back into the fabric, do not lean away from it
*Be careful coming out of this, there is a lot of twisting around with the shoulders and grip
AKA:_____

Entry #2

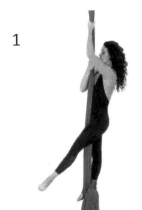

1

Begin from a single foot lock. Reach your left arm up a few inches above your head and grab.

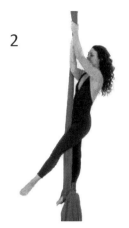

2

Pass your right arm forward between you and the fabric and grab below your left hand.

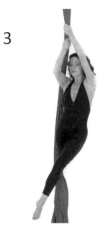

3

Begin to pass your shoulders in front of the fabric, keep your grip the same.

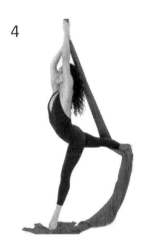

4

Lean your torso forward while maintaining a straight left leg underneath you.

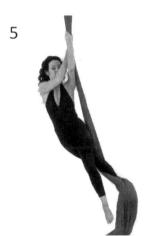

5

Keep your grip the same while you bend your elbows and lean back towards the pole of the fabric.

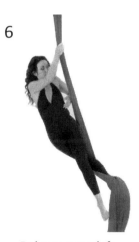

6

Release your left hand and pass your arm back through.

8

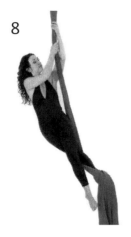

Reach your left hand above your right.

9

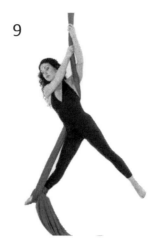

Begin to lean your torso forward and lift your left leg up behind you until the fabric is on your lower back.

10 ★

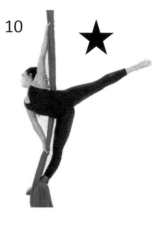

Lift your left leg up into a full arabesque.

11

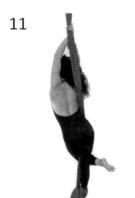

Lower your left leg, cross it in front of your right and spin back the way you came with your left arm up high.

12

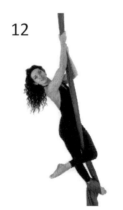

Once you pass your shoulders and head grab the fabric with your right hand below your left.

TIPS
*This is easier than entry #1 on the shoulders and grip
*Step 4 can serve as a pretty line & opportunity for variations with your bottom leg
*Be sure to press your lower back into the fabric during step 10
*The arabesque can be the starting position for many more advanced tricks to come
AKA:_____

Music Box

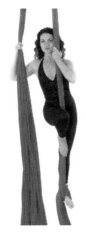

1

Begin from a single foot lock on the left fabric. Hold the tail in your right hand.

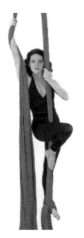

2

Place the tail in your right armpit and circle your right wrist upwards around the fabric once and grab.

3

Lean to the left hooking your right hip crease over the fabric.

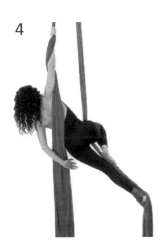

4

Reach behind you with your left arm for the tail.

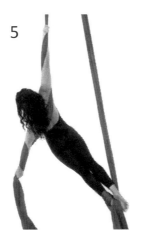

5

Circle your left wrist around the fabric once and join your legs together.

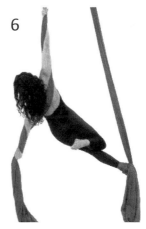

6

Bend your right leg and bring your heel toward your tush keeping your knees together.

7

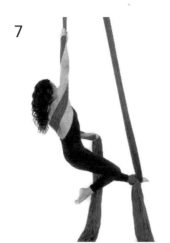

Begin to roll backwards
allowing the fabric to
roll up your left ankle.

8

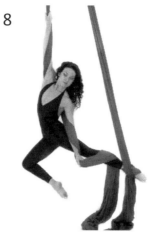

Continue rolling
backwards to complete
one roll.

9

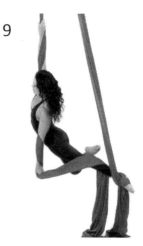

Continue rolling.

10

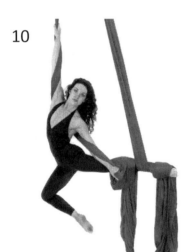

Continue rolling to
complete two rolls.

11

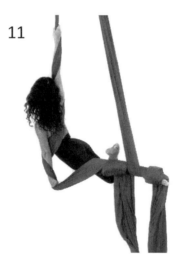

Continue rolling
backwards.

12

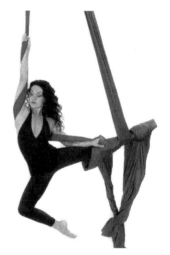

Complete your third
roll.

13

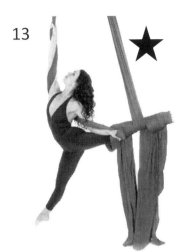

Finish the third roll and straighten your right leg to complete the music box.

14

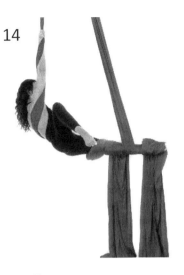

To come out re-trace your path by beginning to unroll the three wraps, lead with your hips.

15

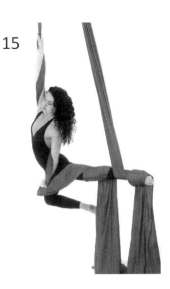

Continue to unroll the third wrap.

16

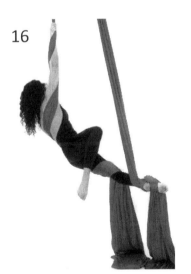

Keep unrolling.

17

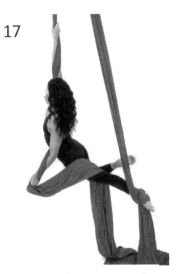

Unroll your second wrap.

18

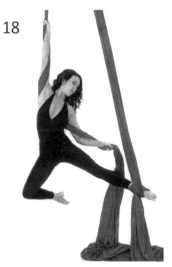

Unroll your first wrap, keep the tail to your left.

19

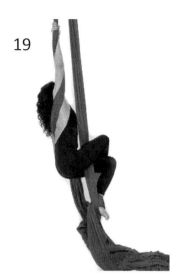

Cross your legs around
the pole of the fabric.

20

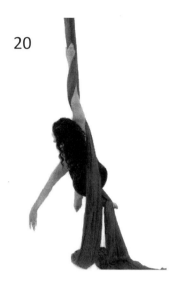

Let go of the tail with
your left hand.

21

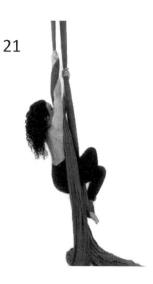

Grab the pole of
the fabric with your
left hand.

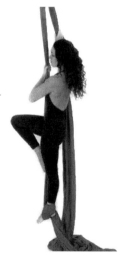

Stand up and
unwind your right
hand.

TIPS
*This move can be strenuous on the grip and
shoulders, be sure to warm up and have a fresh
grip
*Do not just hang from your top arm, instead
pull your shoulder away from your ear to help
engage the latissimus dorsi (lats) for support
*Keep your bottom arm next to your side and
allow the fabric to get twisted during steps 7-13,
it will untwist when you roll out
*If you rolled up 1 time unroll a half turn
*If you rolled up 2 times unroll 1 ½ turns
*If you rolled up 3 times unroll 2 ½ turns
*You can play with different leg variations once
you get comfortable
AKA: _____

Split Roll Up

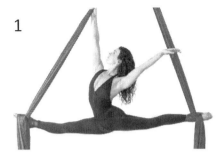

1

Begin from foot lock splits
with your right leg forward.

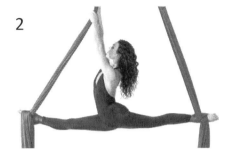

2

Place both hands on the front
fabric.

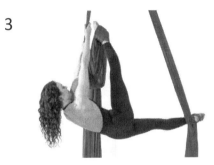

3

Kick your front leg to the right as
you drop your shoulders to the left
to complete the first roll.

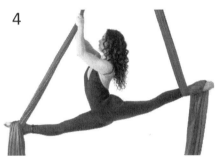

4

You will feel the fabric rolling up
your back ankle. Re-split as low as
you can.

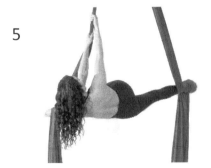

5

Repeat step 3 to complete the
second roll.

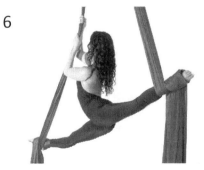

6

Re-split as low as you can.

7

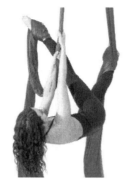

Repeat step 3 to complete your
third roll.

8

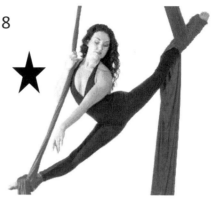

Re-split as low as you can finishing
in a diagonal split. To come out
see page 59 or continue to
Teardrop on page 57.

TIPS
*Having even foot locks is crucial!
*Think of leading the kick (as in step 3) with the pinkie toe side of your foot of the front leg
*If you roll the wrong direction your back foot lock will come undone!
*It can help to move your hands up a few inches in between each roll
*Keep your legs straight to prevent your foot locks from coming loose and possibly falling off during your roll ups
*Three rolls does require hamstring flexibility and hip mobility. If you find three rolls is too much stick with 1-2 for now
AKA: Rotisserie _____

Tear Drop

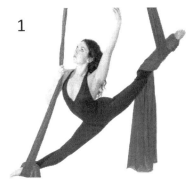

1

Continue from a complete split roll up.

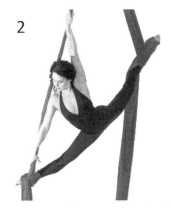

2

Reach your left arm up on the front fabric using a flamenco grip. Once your top hand is secure lower your right hand down with your thumb facing down.

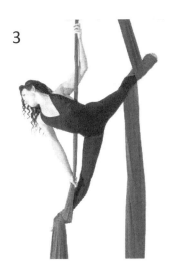

3

Pass your head and shoulders to the front of the fabric. Bend your left elbow securing it on the back of the fabric.

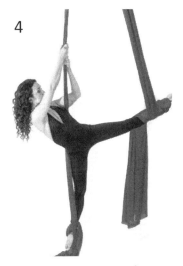

4

Turn your torso to face up joining your right hand with your left. You should feel the fabric on your lower back.

5

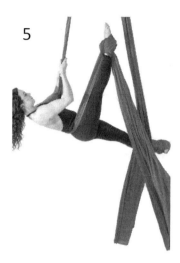

Pull up while lifting your right leg to the side aiming your shin towards the fabric you are holding.

6 ★

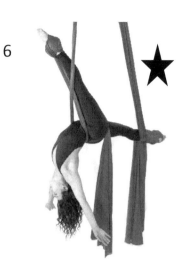

Once your shin is securely pressing into the fabric release your hands.

7

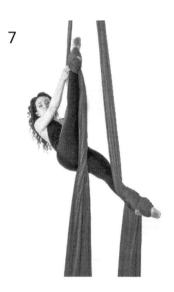

To come out pull up on the fabric that you were just previously holding and release your hooked leg.

8

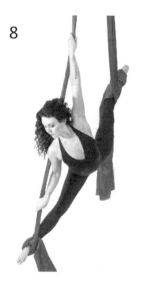

Lower back into a diagonal split. Begin to pass your head and shoulders back the way you came.

10

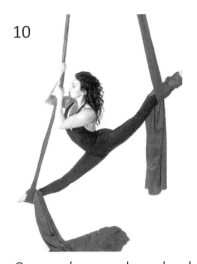

Once you've passed your head and shoulders to the opposite side, move your hands in front of your chest leading with your left (top) hand.

11

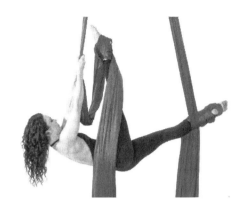

Kick back the way you came by dropping your shoulders to the right and kicking towards the left.

12

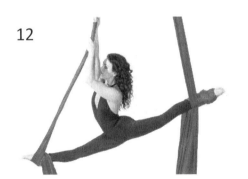

Re-split as low as you can.

13

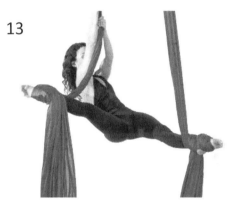

Continue to kick back two more times (for a total of three) to unroll your wrap.

14

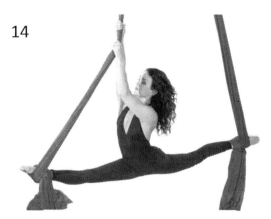

Finish in a split.

TIPS
*Pulling up (step 5) will help to get your shin securely on the fabric
*Do not let go (step 6) unless you feel completely secure
*Be careful when passing your head and shoulders to the front and back of the fabric
*Be sure to ALWAYS move one hand at a time
*When un-rolling, re-split in between each roll to keep your foot locks in place
*Do your best not to kick the opposite fabric when kicking through, doing so may result in your foot lock becoming loose
*Keep your legs straight the entire time! It looks best. Bent legs decrease the tension in your foot locks which may result in them falling off
AKA:_____

Back Spin - Straddle X Back Entry

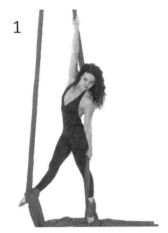

1

Begin from double foot locks with your right leg forward and left leg back. Reach your right arm up on the fabric behind you with your thumb up and left arm down with your thumb pointing down.

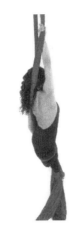

2

Begin to spin backwards towards your left shoulder while joining your legs together and sitting your hips back. Keep the fabric behind you.

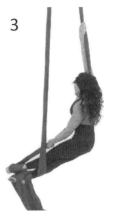

3

Continue to turn until you can easily place your right elbow on the back side of the fabric that is behind you.

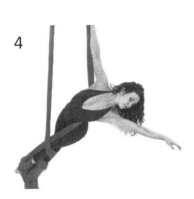

4

Keeping your legs together reach out with your left arm until you feel the fabric slide down to your lower back.

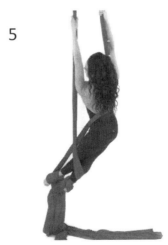

5

Keep your right hand secure where it is. Reach your left arm across to the left fabric.

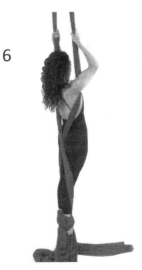

6

Stand straight up, you will have an X behind your back.

7

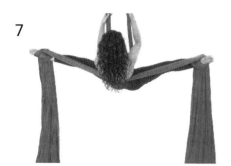

Straddle your legs directly to the side while pressing the fabric forward and lean your shoulders back.

8

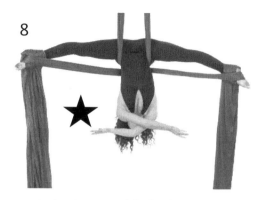

Arrive in a straddle back position.

9

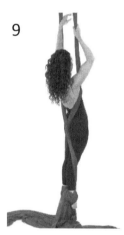

To come out join your legs together underneath and place your hands on the right side.

10

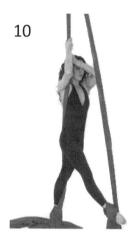

Bring your torso out in between both fabrics.

11

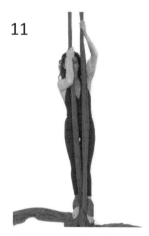

Using one hand at a time grab each fabric to come out of the X.

TIPS

*This can be confusing! Pay attention to the set up in step 1, which leg and arm go where
*When doing the back spin movement (steps 2-3) keep the fabric behind you, it is easy to get mixed up and inadvertently bring it to the front
*Try the same method on your other side
AKA:_____

The Pin Up - Straddle X Back Entry

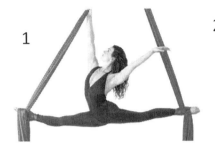

1

Begin from double foot lock splits on the right.

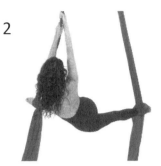

2

Continue the movement and join your ankles together.

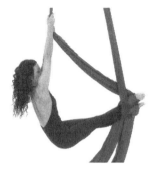

3

Drop your shoulders to the left allowing your legs to make a scissor shape.

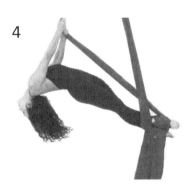

4

Press your hips up and arch your upper back.

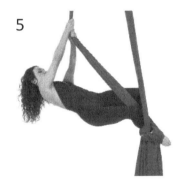

5

Turn to the right and bend your knees.

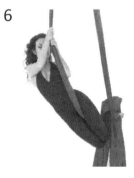

6

Scoop the fabric up in between your knees and continue to turn to the right.

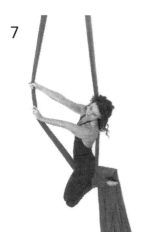

7

Press the front fabric forward while pressing your back into the fabric behind you creating the "pin up" pose.

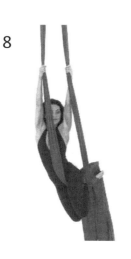

8

Reach your right arm up higher on the right fabric. Lean your shoulders back in between the fabrics and grab the left piece.

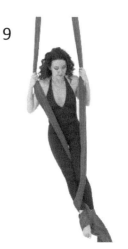

9

Pull up, straighten your right leg and begin to bend your left keeping your knees together.

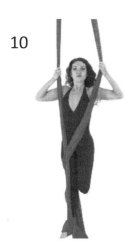

10

Keep the X open in front of you.

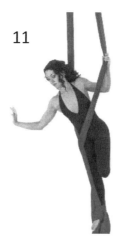

11

Reach your right arm forward in between the X and bring your shoulders through.

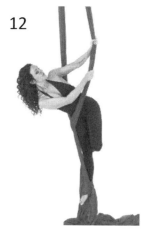

12

Slightly turn towards the left, grab the fabric with your right hand.

13

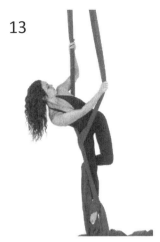

Place your left hand
on the left fabric.

14

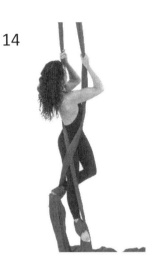

Come to an upright
position and begin to
turn your torso
forward.

15

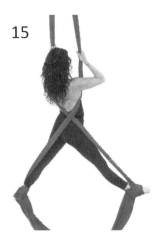

Straighten your legs
into a low straddle and
turn your torso
completely forward
until you feel an X on
your back.

16

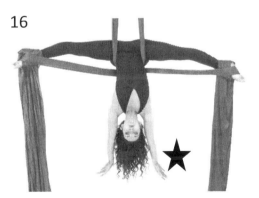

Invert into a straddle.

17

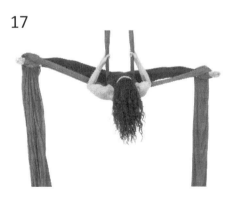

To come out grab the fabrics and
re-trace your path.

18

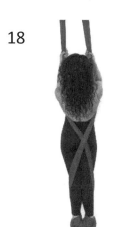

Join your legs together underneath you.

19

Grab the fabric that is closest to your back →

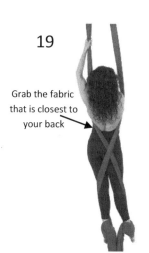

Grab the fabric with your left hand and reach your right arm in between.

20

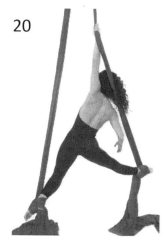

Open into a right split keeping your left hand on the fabric. You will end up in a flamenco grip with your left hand.

21

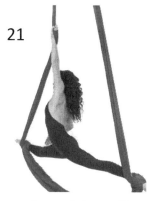

Lower into a split.

22

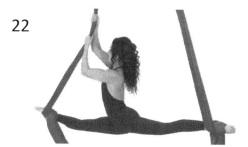

Place your right hand on the front fabric, carefully take your left hand off and place it under your right hand.

TIPS
*Be precise in step 5, scooping the fabric between your knees can be a challenge when learning
*Keep your ankles equally together during steps 3-8
*This is called "Pin Up" for the position made in step 7 on pg. 64, it somewhat resembles a pin up girl
*Always grab the fabric that is closest to your back when exiting
AKA:_____

Uneven Foot Locks – Aerial Chair

1
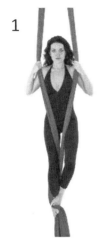

Begin from a classic climb with open fabrics.

2
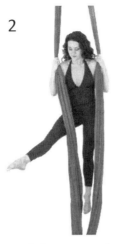

Release your feet preparing to wrap your right leg.

3
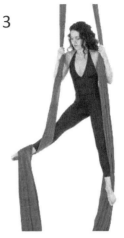

Wrap your right leg outside around the right fabric.

4
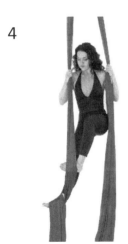

Begin wrapping a single foot lock using the outside of your left foot.

5
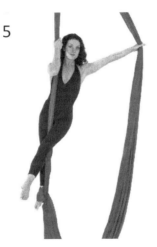

Complete your right foot lock. Hold the free fabric in your left hand.

6
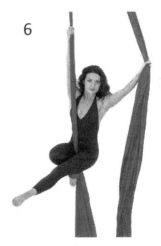

Squat down on your right.

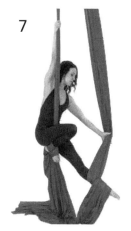

7

Wrap your left leg around the free fabric from the outside in. Pull up approx. 1 foot of fabric.

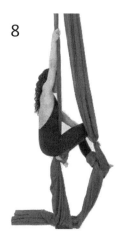

8

Reach the fabric across the top of your foot.

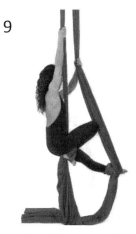

9

Complete your foot lock on the left.

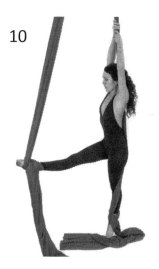

10

Stand up and place your back side against the foot locked fabric that is closer to the floor.

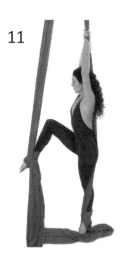

11

Bend your front knee to point up.

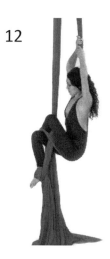

12

Pull up while crossing your left leg (back leg) over your front bent leg. Keep the fabric in the middle of your back and tush.

13

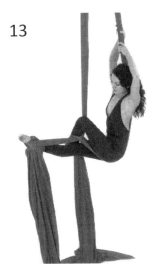

Straighten your
bottom leg.

14 ★

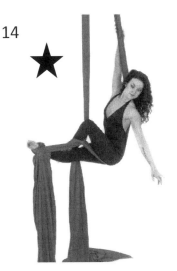

Arrive in your aerial chair. Option
to reach one arm off or choose
another choreographic position
with your arms.

Optional Variation

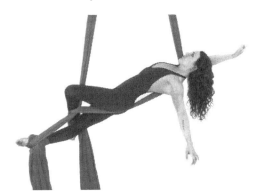

Press your hips up and reach your right arm
back. Keep the fabric in the middle of your tush
and to the right of your neck.

15

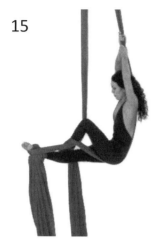

To come out grab the
fabric behind you with
both hands.

16

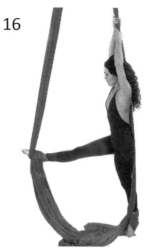

Pull up and uncross
your legs. Take one
foot lock off at a
time.

TIPS
*Always lean your back side against the fabric with a lower foot lock
*Keep the fabric in the middle of your tush and back the entire time, it
can easily slip to the side (see step 12)
*This is a great resting pose!
AKA: _____

**"Many of life's failures are experienced by people who did not realize
how close they were to success when they gave up."**
Thomas Edison

WRAPS & TRICKS

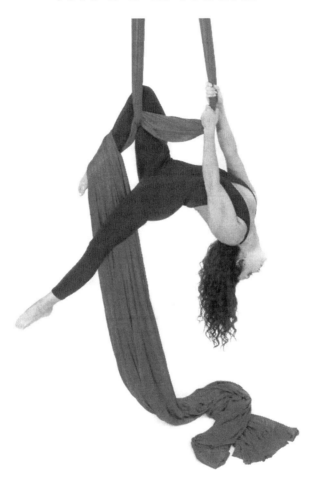

Cross Back into Stag

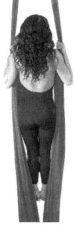

1

Begin suspended on your arms in between the fabrics.

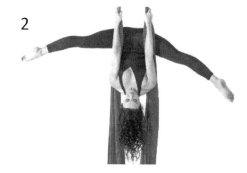

2

Invert into a straddle.

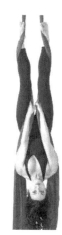

3

Crochet your feet around the fabrics from the outside in. Press your arches into the fabric, point your feet and sickle inwards.

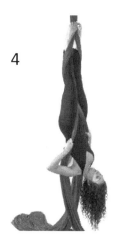

4

Squeeze your legs and feet together while you slide your hands down towards your hips.

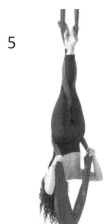

5

Continue to slide your hands until you are holding the fabrics a few inches behind your back.

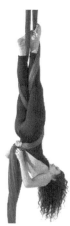

6

Carefully cross the fabrics behind your back.

7

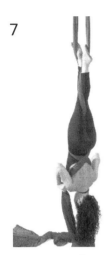

Once you have the opposing fabric in each hand slide your hands down the fabric until your hands are in front of your armpits.

8

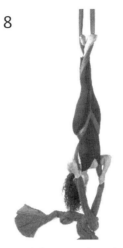

Using one hand at a time flip your grip the opposite direction so your thumbs point down.

9

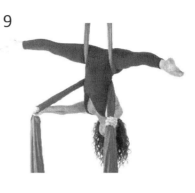

Extend your legs into a straddle and straighten your arms out in front of you in a V shape.

11

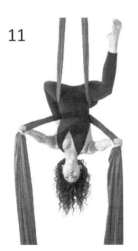

Bend your legs into a double stag position.

10

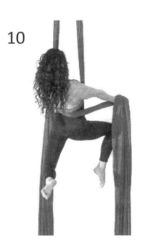

Lower your legs and begin to lift your chest up while keeping your arms straight in a V shape in front of you.

12

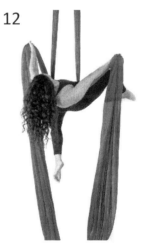

Arrive upright.

13

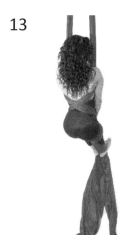

Place the fabrics in between your legs and step for a classic climb.

14

Grab the fabric that is closer to your back

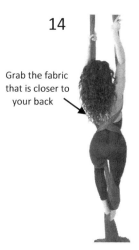

Keep your feet in a secure climb as you reach your arms up.

15

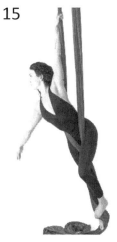

Place your left hand on the left fabric and reach your right arm through the middle.

16

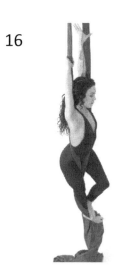

Sneak your shoulders back in between the fabrics one at a time.

17

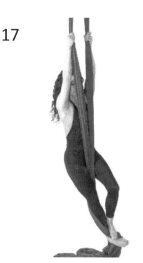

End with the fabrics in front of you.

Crocheted Foot

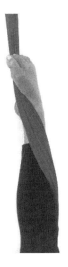

When crocheting your feet around the fabric, your feet need to be pointed and sickled in. Normally a sickled foot is incorrect but in this case, it is used as a lever.

Option- Single Leg Crochet

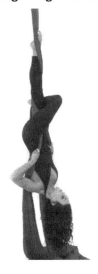

Instead of wrapping both feet around either fabric you can choose the single leg variation. One foot is crocheted around both fabrics and the opposite leg is bent and crossed over.

TIPS

*When crocheting your feet upwards (see step 3, pg. 72) be aware of not losing height. Circle the leg up and around the fabric, do not allow yourself to sink down

*Try the entire sequence off the ground first before attempting it in the air

*Sickling your feet around the fabric is necessary for safety during steps 3-8 (see page 72-73)

*The cross behind your back can be challenging, always have a crash mat and spotter when learning

*When you flip your grip the opposite direction (see step 8 pg. 73) keep your legs and feet squeezing together or you will slide!

*The first steps (1-5) are the beginning to many other tricks

*Wrapping 2 knots behind you (step 6 pg. 72) is necessary for some advanced tricks

AKA: Tick-tack

Hip Key - Secretary

1

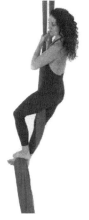

Begin from a classic
climb with the fabrics
open.

2

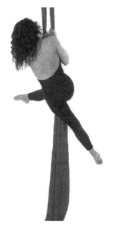

Release your feet, scissor
your legs with your right
leg forward and left leg
back into a hip key.

3

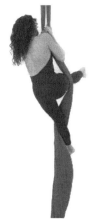

Place the tail in
between your legs.

4

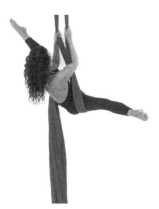

Pass through a straddle
aiming your left leg up.

5

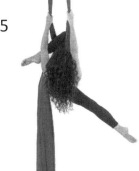

Keep the fabrics open,
bend your left knee
and pass it between
the fabrics. Enter in the
opening that is closer
to you.

6

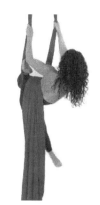

Continue to pass your
knee until your foot
clears.

7

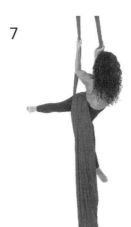

Flip the grip on your
right hand so your
thumb points down.

8

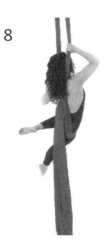

Place the fabric in
your right hand
behind you.

9

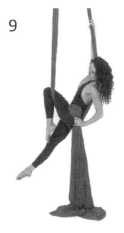

Turn your torso slightly
left to sit on the fabric
place it in the center of
your back and tush. Hold
the tail in your left hand if
you are slipping.

10 ★

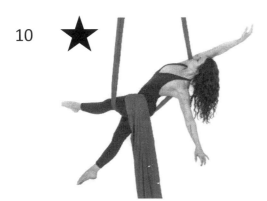

Press your hips up, straighten your legs
and reach your arms out placing the
fabric just to the right of your neck.

11

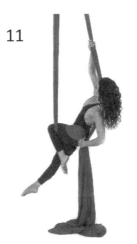

To come out return to a
sitting position.

12

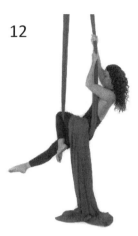

Pass your head and shoulders to the right. Grab the fabric that was behind you with both hands.

13

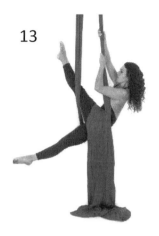

Lift your left leg up in between the fabrics.

14

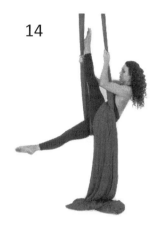

The moment your left leg clears the fabric reach your right arm across and grab the right side.

15

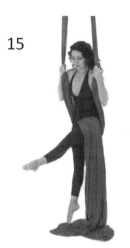

End in between the fabrics.

16

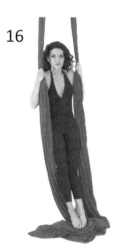

Pull up and lower your left leg down.

TIPS

*You must have a solid hip key before attempting this trick

*It is crucial to lift your left leg up high (see step 4 pg. 76) to ensure the fabric falls to your hip

*Place your knee in the gap that is closer to you (step 5), if you place it incorrectly it will be challenging to slide the fabric behind your back

*Keep the fabrics open the entire time

*Pressing your hips up versus sitting will prevent you from slipping

AKA:_____

Knee Tangle

1

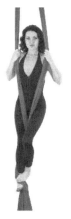

Begin from a classic climb in between the fabrics.

2

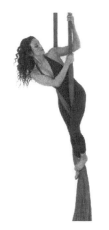

Bring your torso in between, place both hands on the left.

3

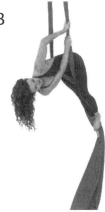

Lean forward.

4

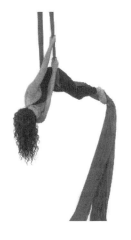

Continue to press your feet together and lift your heels up behind you.

5

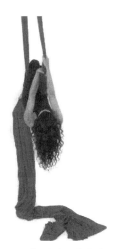

When you feel the fabric move below your hip bones turn to the left and bend both knees until you face up.

6

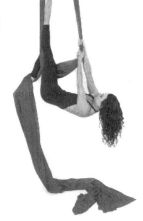

The fabric will be "tangled" just above your right knee. Keep your right leg bent and take your left leg out.

7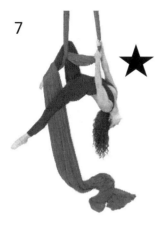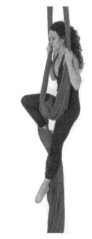

Lower your left leg behind you and arch your upper back to complete the knee tangle position.

8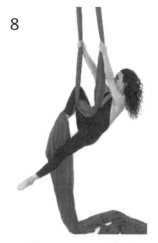

To come out climb above your knee.

9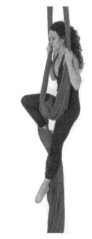

Continue climbing above until the wrap loosens around your right leg.

10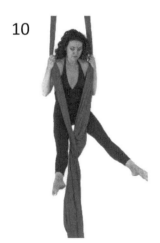

Lengthen your legs.

11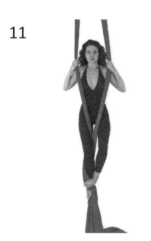

Re-wrap your feet in the classic climb.

TIPS
*Think of your body as a plank from your waist down during steps 2-4
*Keep your right leg bent (step 5-7) if you straighten your right leg, or your leg drops away from your body "knee tangle" will fall off
*Try it on your other side, If you are on a right side climb grab the left fabric & vice versa
AKA:_____

Creature

1
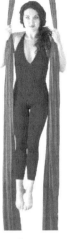

Begin in between the fabrics suspended on your arms.

2
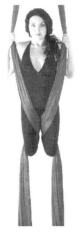

Circle your legs around the fabrics from the outside in, bring your heels towards your tush.

3
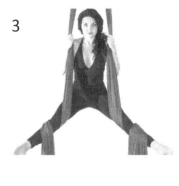

Extend your legs to the side in a low straddle.

4
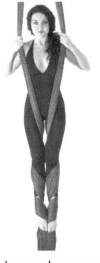

Circle your legs around one more time to complete two wraps.
(this is the same as the double foot lock wrap)

5
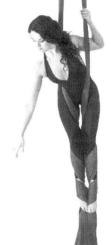

Squeeze your legs and feet together, reach one arm between the fabrics.

6
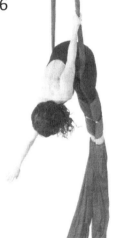

Lean forward in a pike.

7

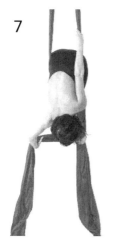

Grab the tail in one hand with your knuckles facing down.

8

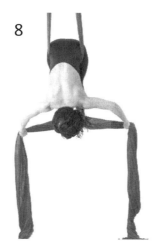

Once your grip is secure reach for the other tail.

9

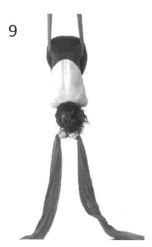

Roll the fabrics around your wrists once and press your knuckles forward.

(this gives you extra leverage for the next steps)

10

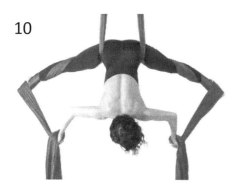

Straddle your legs directly to the side allowing the fabric to slide below your hip bones.

11

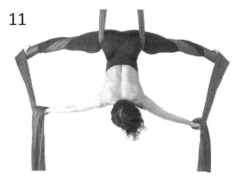

Begin to roll your pelvis upwards while pulling your legs over your head.

12

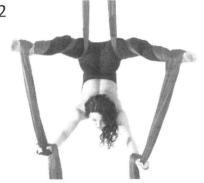

Continue to pull your legs over while rotating your shoulders and hips until you see your feet over your head.

13

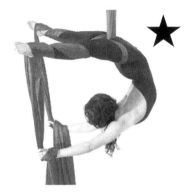

Pull down on the fabric to secure your position.

14

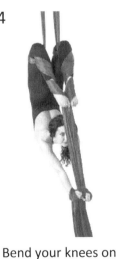

Bend your knees on the outside of the pole of the fabric and bring your feet towards your head.
(if you miss steps 12-13 bend your knees right away and you will end up here)

15

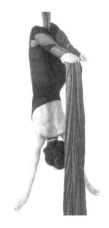

Release the tails.

16

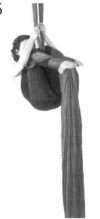

Sit up and grab the fabrics above your knees.

17

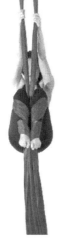

Climb above your
knees.

18

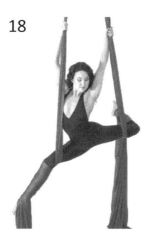

Open your legs into a
stag position.
Option: Open into a
straddle.

19

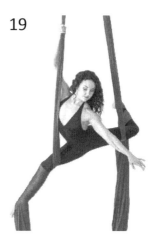

Reach one arm
forward.

20

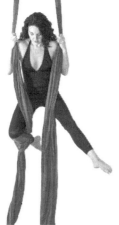

Pull up and gracefully
unwind your legs.

21

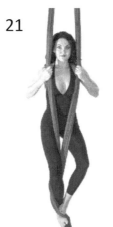

Step on the fabric
in your classic
climb.

TIPS
*This requires hip and
shoulder mobility as well as
hamstring and back flexibility
*The grip in step 9 (see pg.
82) is optional, you can
simply hold the fabric, this
version gives you more
leverage to pull your legs
over your head
*The closer in your grab the
tails the more challenging
this is on your flexibility
*In some cases achieving
step 12 (see pg. 83) will be
challenging, try going from
step 11 directly to step 14 by
bending your knees outside
of the fabrics
AKA: Scorpion

Back Balance into Flag

1

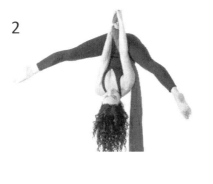

Begin from a classic climb on the right.

2

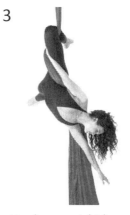

Invert in a straddle on the right.

3

Hook your right knee above your hands. Release your left hand and swim (reach back) for the tail.

4

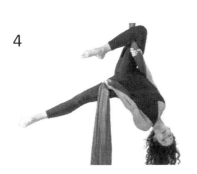

Grab the tail with your palm facing up. Press your left arm into your side creating a shelf across your lower back.

5

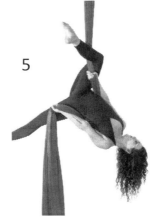

Begin to unhook your right knee, continue to press your left arm into your side.

6

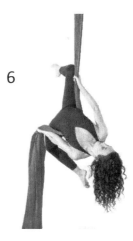

Keep your hips facing up as you release your right leg.

7

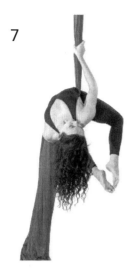

Arch your upper back and meet your legs in a diamond shape.

8

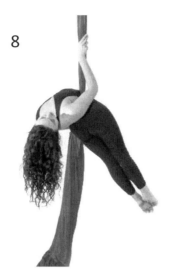

Option: Lengthen your legs and join them together.

9 ★

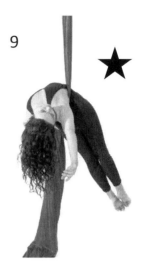

Option: Once you find your balance, reach your right arm back.

10

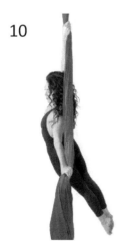

To begin the flag, reach your right arm up high and continue to hold the tail in your left.

11

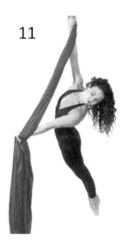

Circle your left arm around to the front creating a "flag."

12

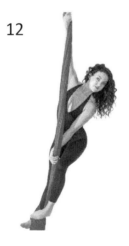

Step on the fabric in your classic climb.

13

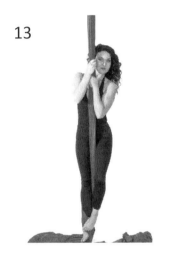

Move your hands in
front of your chest
one at a time.

TIPS
*When practicing try the maneuver on the
floor instead of in the air and skip the flag.
Just step down instead
*You can easily flip to the side, if you are
not in proper position. ALWAYS have a
crash mat and spotter when learning
*The oppositional pull of pressing your left
arm forward and pulling your right shoulder
back will help you find your balance
*Having your legs in a diamond shape (step
7) is easier than legs together (step 8)
*There are other tricks you can eventually
do from a back balance, the flag is just one!
AKA: _____

**"Never stop doing your best just because someone
doesn't give you credit."**
Unknown

Single Ankle Hang

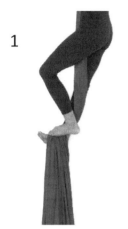

1

Begin from a classic climb.

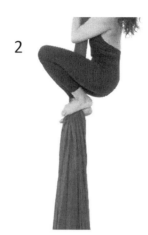

2

Squat down with the fabric in between your legs.

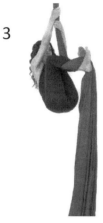

3

Lean back keeping the fabric draped over your right foot.

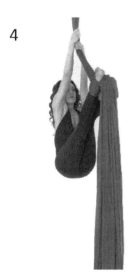

4

Turn your right foot inwards and firmly flex placing the pole of the fabric over the top of your foot.

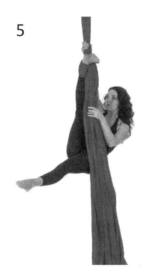

5

Continue to firmly flex your foot and walk your hands down the tail.

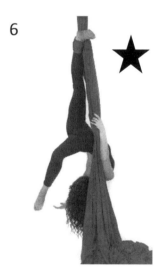

6

Arch back and hang from your ankle.

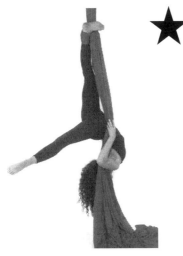

Option: Extend your leg behind you in an arabesque.

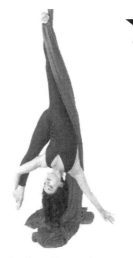

Option: Extend your leg to the side.

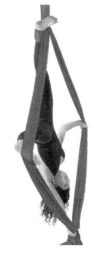

Option: Create a box!

9

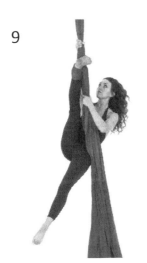

To come out keep the tail to the left, sit up and begin to climb up the tail.

10

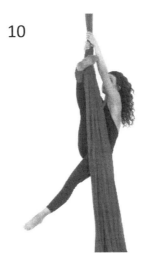

Keep climbing until you reach to the pole of the fabric above your foot.

11

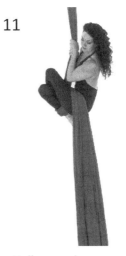

Pull up and cross your left leg over your right. Straighten your legs and the fabric will fall off.

CORRECT Foot Position
Fabric is on the outside of the foot

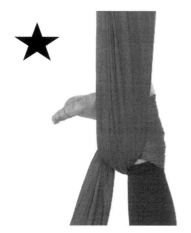

INCORRECT Foot Position
Fabric is on the inside of the foot

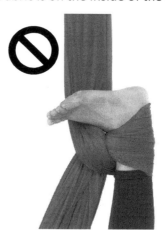

TIPS
*You MUST firmly flex your foot the entire time or you may fall
*Wearing full ankle length leggings will be beneficial, bare lower legs may result in the fabric sticking to you especially during steps 3-5 (pg. 88)
*There are numerous shapes you can make within the single ankle hang, get creative!
*Keep track of the tail when coming out. If you did a single ankle hang on the right the tail needs to be on your left when climbing up. If you cross it over to the opposite side you will get tangled when coming out!
AKA: _____

Scorpion

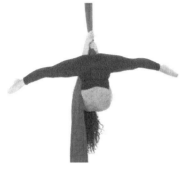

1

Invert in a straddle with the fabric on your right.

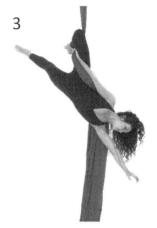

2

Hook your right knee above your hands.

3

Release your left hand and swim (reach back) for the tail.

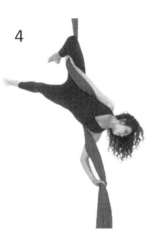

4

Grab the tail with your thumb facing up.

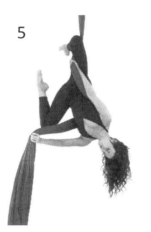

5

Bend your left knee.

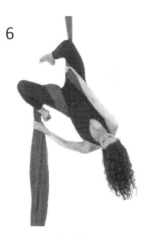

6

Wrap the fabric over your knee from the inside, pull the fabric over the top of your foot to complete a single thigh wrap.

7

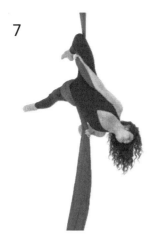

Slide your hand
down the tail.

8

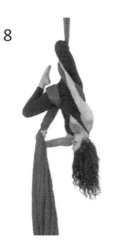

Repeat steps 5-7 to
create a 2nd wrap.

9

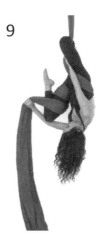

Repeat steps 5-7 to
create a 3rd wrap.

10

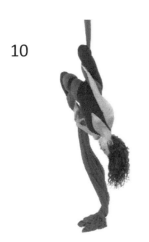

Place the fabric over
the top of your left
foot, hold the tail in
your left hand.

11

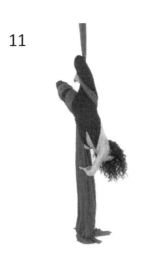

Release your right hand
and reach for the tail
over your head.

12

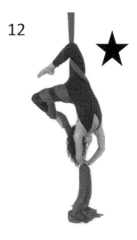

Rotate your left leg
behind you and pull on
the tail bringing your
foot towards your head.

13

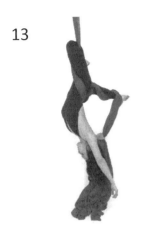

Extend your left leg
behind you.

14

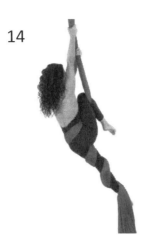

Sit up and reach your
arms high above
your knee.

15

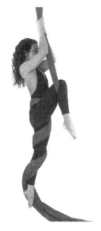

Pull up.

16

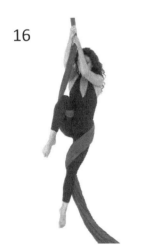

Allow the tail to unwind
off of your left leg.

17

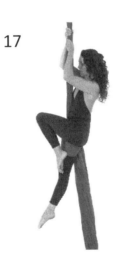

Once all three wraps
are off you will end up
in a thigh hitch.

18

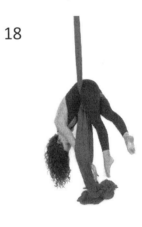

Drop your torso to the
right and swim the tail
behind your back with
your left arm.

19

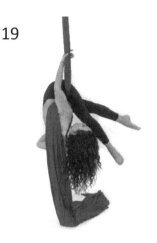

Once the tail is behind your back, reach your hands up to the pole end. Pull up and the fabric will fall off your waist.

TIPS
*Climb at least 2 climbs up so you have enough tail to work with
*Wrap the fabric over your knee (see step 5-6, pg. 91) versus trying to toss it over your foot, this is a common mistake
*Allow the fabric to slide through your hand during steps 4-10 if you completely let go, the fabric will most likely get messy and become hard to manage
*Steps 3-7 create a single thigh wrap (aka "Catchers") which is a commonly used wrap for many tricks
AKA: Gazelle, Stag, Catchers Lock Wrap

_____

Flamingo

1

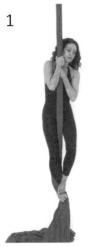

Begin from a right side climb.

2

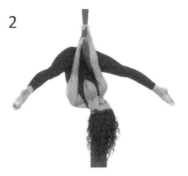

Invert with the fabric on your right.

3

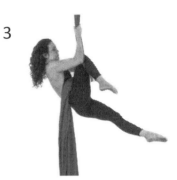

Hook your right knee above your hands and climb above your knee.

4

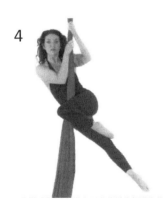

Pull up and press your hips forward feel the fabric around your right leg slide up as high as possible into a thigh hitch.

5

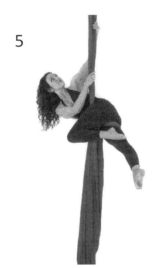

Find the center of the fabric with your left hand.

6

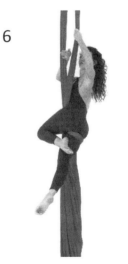

Reach your right arm through the center.

7

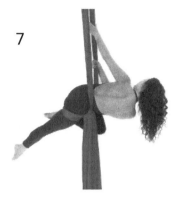

Keep reaching and
pass your torso
through the center.

8

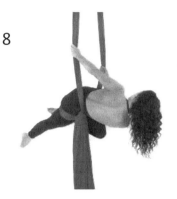

Turn onto your back.
Option: Turn and sit on
the fabric to end up in
an aerial chair (see step
14 pg. 97).

9

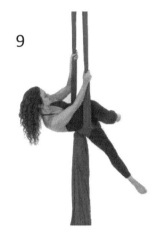

10

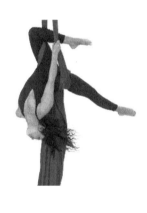

Hook your left leg
around the left fabric
from the outside in.

11

Once the left leg is
secure, arch back.

12 ★

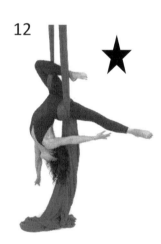

Create a nice line with
your arms.

13

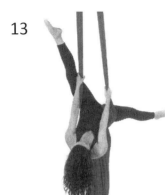

To come out reach up,
grab the fabrics and
un hook your left leg.

14

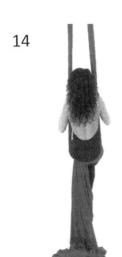

Pull up, press the
fabric down and sit
on the fabric. This is
your aerial seat.
(the aerial seat is the base for
other tricks to come)

15

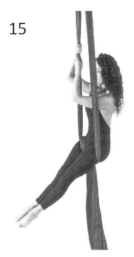

To come out start by
placing both hands
on the right side.

16

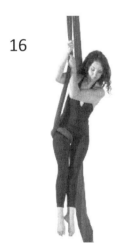

Bring your torso
forward in between
the fabrics until you
feel the fabric slide off
your tush.

17

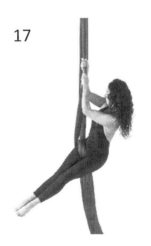

Begin a turn to the
right.

18

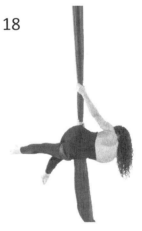

Continue to turn to the
right until your top hip
presses into the pole of
the fabric.

19

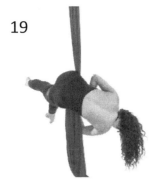

Release your hands.

20

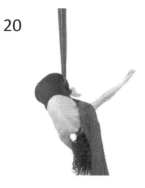

Swim the fabric
behind your back
with your left arm.

21

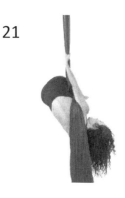

Grab the pole of the
fabric with your left
hand.

22

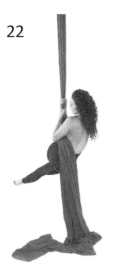

Grab the fabric with
your right hand and
pull up.

23

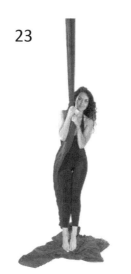

Lower your legs down
and the fabric will fall
off your waist.

TIPS

*It is crucial that you
press your hips forward
(step 4 pg. 95) so the
fabric slides up high on
your thigh

*Sometimes finding the
center of the fabric is a
challenge, looking up
towards the top of the
fabric can be helpful to
find the separation

*The aerial chair (step
14 pg. 97) is the base
for tricks to come!

*Option to skip steps 9-
13 and go straight to
the aerial seat

AKA: _____

Mermaid

1

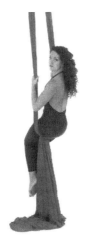

Begin from the aerial seat (see page 97).

2

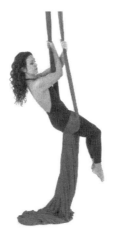

Cross your left arm over the front of the fabric and grab the right side. Reach your right arm behind to grab the left.

3

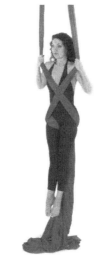

Pull the fabrics apart to make an X.

4

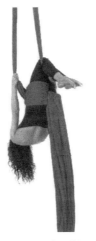

Invert into a pike.

5

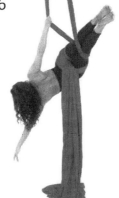

Hook the back of both knees over the fabric on your left side.

6

Hold the fabric with your right hand and release your left. Join your legs together and press your hips forward.

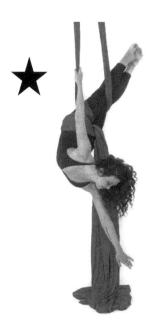

7

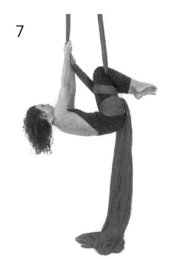

To come out bend
both knees and place
your left hand next to
your right.

8

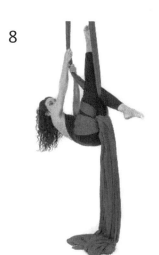

Unhook your right
leg.

9

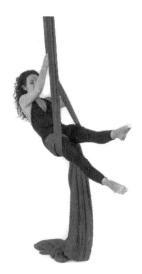

Unhook your left
leg.

10

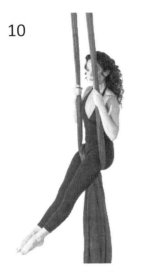

Place your hands on the left fabric and end in the aerial seat. To come out see page 97-98 or continue onto Cupid, the next trick.

To come out see page 97-98

TIPS

*Steps 4-5 (pg. 99) take a lot of strength! Make sure your hands are shoulder height and elbows are into your sides

*Going through a tuck versus a pike (in step 4) is easier

*You can play with leg variations once in position, bend one leg, straighten the other, or bend both and reach your feet towards your head

*The height of your right hand (step 5) determines the shape of your "mermaid" if your hand is higher you won't make as much of a J shape, instead you will be more horizontal

AKA:_____

"Perfection is not attainable, but if we chase perfection we can catch excellence."

Vince Lombardi

Cupid

1

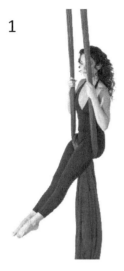

Begin from the aerial
seat (see pg. 97).

2

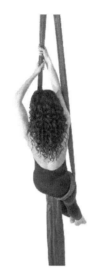

Place both hands on
the left fabric.

3

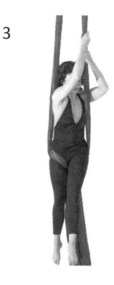

Bring your torso and
tush forward.

4

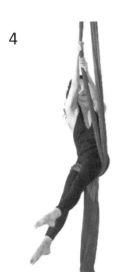

Continue forward until
the right and left fabric
come close together.

5

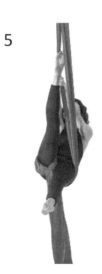

Keep your hands on
the left side and lift
your right leg up in
between the opening.

6

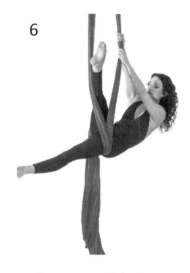

Lower your right leg
towards the left.

7

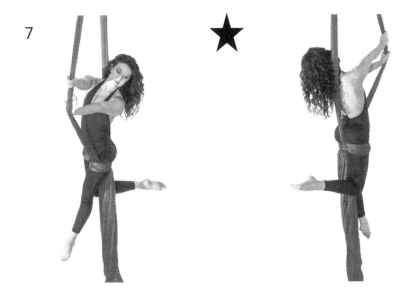

Aim your right leg down while you press the fabric
forward creating a "bow and arrow" shape.

8

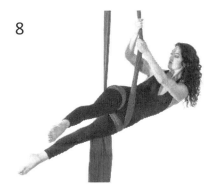

To come out begin by dropping
your torso to the left.

9

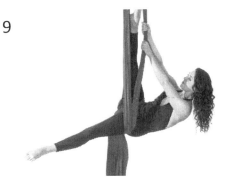

Lift your right leg up and the
direction way you came in
between the fabrics.

10

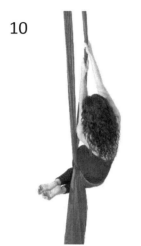

Meet your legs together and bend your knees.

11

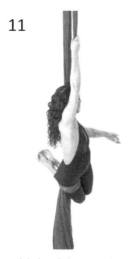

Hold the fabric with your right hand and release your left bringing your left arm in front of the fabric you are holding.

12

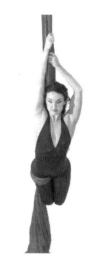

Pass your shoulders to the front and place your left hand below your right.

13

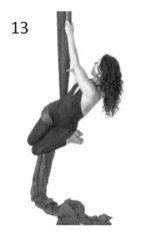

Continue to turn around the fabric.

14

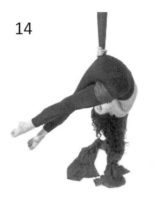

End with your right shoulder aiming down in a thigh hitch on the right. Swim the fabric behind your back with your left arm.

TIPS
*This trick is known to pinch your inner thigh, not everything is aerial is comfortable!
*Steps 4-6 (pg. 102) can feel awkward and require hamstring flexibility
*The flamingo, mermaid and cupid can be linked together to create one sequence
AKA:_____

S-Wrap - Flamenco Entry

1

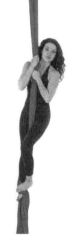

Begin from a classic
climb on the right.

2

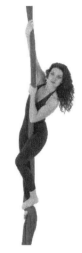

Reach your right arm up
and around the fabric
using a flamenco grip.

3

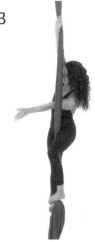

Pass your left arm forward
in the space between you
and the fabric.

4

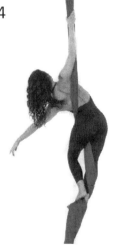

Continue reaching your
left arm forward until
the fabric is behind
your back.

5

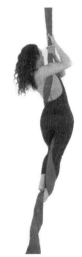

Lower your right hand
down and meet your
left hand next to it.

6

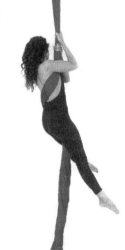

Keep the tail to the
outside of your left hip
as you release your feet
from the fabric.

7

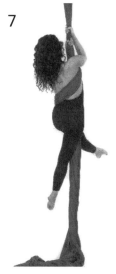

Scissor your legs passing the tail towards your right hip.

8

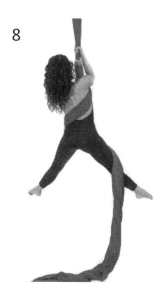

Open your right leg to the side.

9

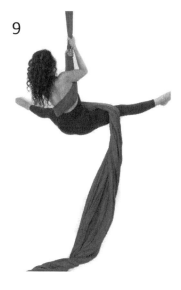

Straddle, keep the tail to your right.

10

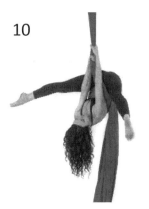

Invert into a straddle.

11

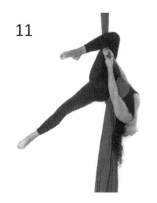

Hook your right knee above your hands and turn your left leg behind you.

12

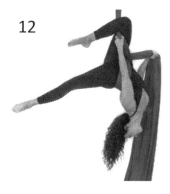

Release your right hand and grab the tail.

13

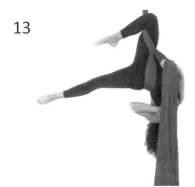

Pass the tail in front of your body across your waist and towards your left hip.

14

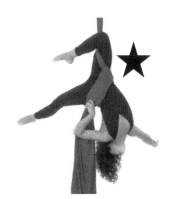

Arrive in your S-Wrap. Continue to Windmill (pg. 112 & 114) or come out.

15

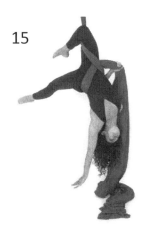

To come out pass the tail to your right side using your right hand.

16

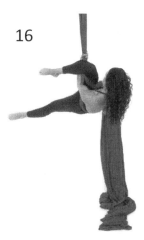

Reach up and under your left knee with your left hand.

17

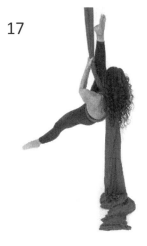

Unhook your right leg, continue holding the tail in your right hand and pull it tightly to your right.

18

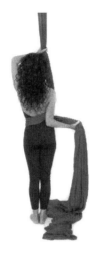

Step down.

"Until you spread your wings, you'll have no idea how far you can fly."
Unknown

S-Wrap - Single Thigh Wrap Entry

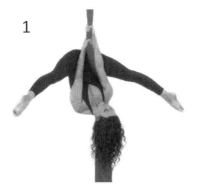

1

Begin from a straddle
inversion on the right.

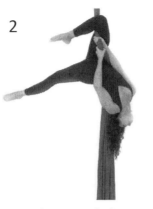

2

Hook your right knee
above your hands and
turn your left leg
behind you.

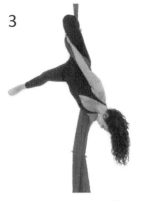

3

Swim (reach back) for
the fabric with your left
hand, grab the tail with
your thumb facing up.

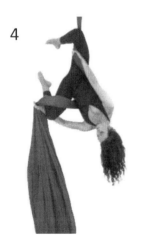

4

Bend your left knee
and wrap your left
thigh from the inside.

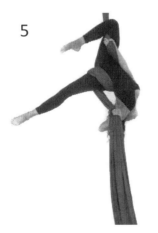

5

Pull the tail over your
knee and foot, extend
your left leg behind you.

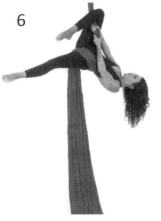

6

Release the tail and
place your left hand
under your right.

7

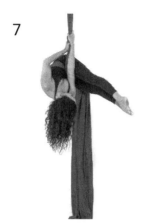

Unhook your right leg and pike both legs to the right behind the pole of the fabric into a meat hook (see pg. 123).

8

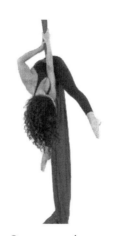

Open your legs dropping the tail off in between them.

9

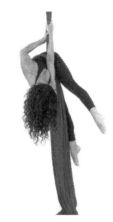

Go around the tail with your right leg.

10

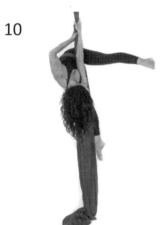

Place the tail on your right hip.

11

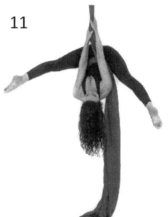

Open into a straddle.

12

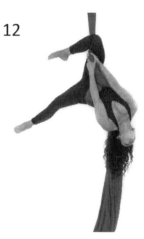

Hook your right knee above your hands and turn your left leg behind you.

13

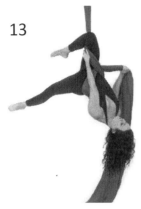

Grab the tail with
your right hand.

14

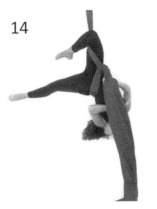

Pass the tail to the front,
across your waist and
towards your left hip.

15

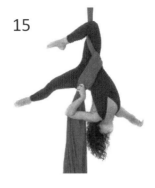

Arrive in your S-Wrap.
Continue to Windmill
(see pg. 112 & 114) or
come out (see pg.
107-108).

TIPS
*You have to be experienced with a meat hook to attempt this (see pg. 123)
*Keep your hands in the same position during steps 6-12, it is tempting to move your left hand higher to lessen the effort on your obliques. If you do this your hands will be too high when you go to hook your knee for step 12
*The S-Wrap is the base for windmills and star drops
*There are several different ways to get into the S-Wrap!
AKA: _____

Windmill with Diamond Legs

1

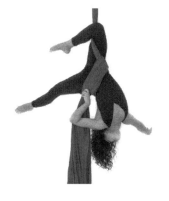

Begin from a S-Wrap.

2

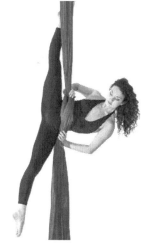

Turn your body sideways, open your legs into a straddle and press your top foot on pole of the fabric.

3

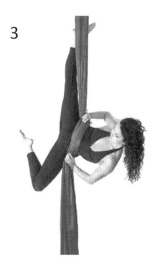

Bend your bottom leg. Press your right hand into the knot and your left hand into the tail across your waist.

4

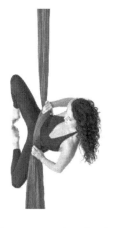

Release your top foot and meet your toes together with your legs in a diamond shape.

5

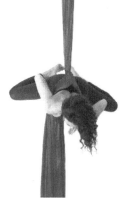

Rotate a quarter turn to face down, pressing your right hand into the tail next to your right hip. Keep your body in the same shape as step 4.

6

Turn a quarter turn to the side, place your left hand on the opposite side of the knot.

7

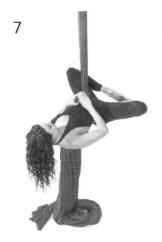

Make a quarter turn to face up pressing your hands into the knot. Repeat steps 4-6 to continue multiple rotations.

8

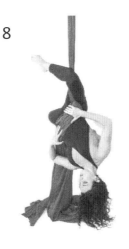

Lean back and hook your right leg.

9

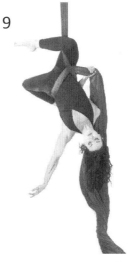

To come out pass the tail to your right using your right hand.

10

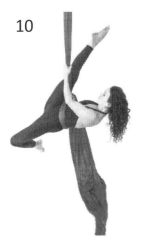

Reach up under your left knee with your left hand, unhook your knee, hold the tail with your right.

11

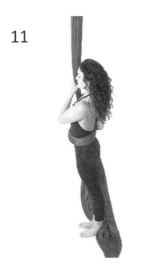

Pull the tail to the right as you step down.

TIPS
*Use the palm of your hands to help you to rotate within the knot, do not use your fingers or they may get stuck!
*Keep your body in the same shape during steps 4-7, if you collapse or bring your knees together, the fabric will cinch up around your waist and become very tight
*It requires core, back and glute strength to maintain your position AKA: Wheel Down

Windmill

1

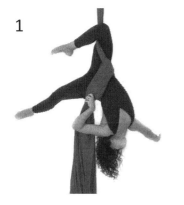

Begin from a S-Wrap.

2

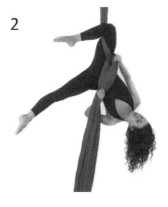

Extend your bottom leg in a straddle to the side.

3

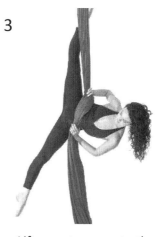

Lift your torso up to the side and extend your top leg to a straddle.
Option: Hook your right foot on the top fabric to prepare.

4

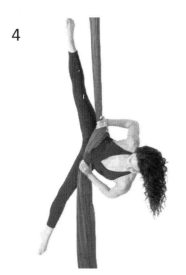

Release your top foot from the fabric maintaining your same body position.

5

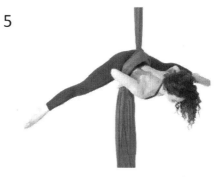

Rotate a quarter turn to face down, pressing your right hand into the tail next to your right hip. Keep your body in the same shape as step 4.

6

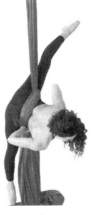

Make another quarter turn to the right. Release your left hand and continue pressing your right hand into the tail.

7

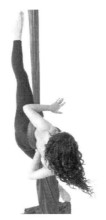

Release your left hand, place to the left of the knot.

8

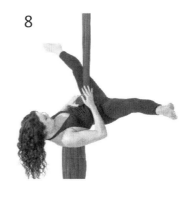

Complete one more quarter turn to face upward. Press your hands into the knot to stop your movement. To continue rotations repeat steps 4-8.

9

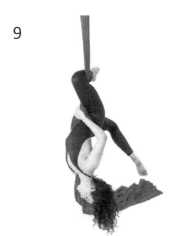

Lean back and hook your right leg. To come out see pg. 107-108.

TIPS

*This requires a lot of core strength to maintain the same body shape as you turn. Keep your abs engaged, lower back lengthening, legs turned out and tight the entire time!

*Going from step 4-5 can be a challenge, if you collapse and lose your shape the fabric will cinch up around your stomach, the goal is to keep it on your hips

*Going slowly in quarter turns will help you to understand the movement, hand work and body position. Once you have the hang of it you can speed it up

*The straddle legs are more challenging than the diamond leg variation

*The ceiling height factors in how many rotations you can do, if it's 12-14 feet you can do 2, 15-20 feet 3-4. The higher the ceiling, the more rotations!

AKA: Wheel Down _____

CONDITIONING

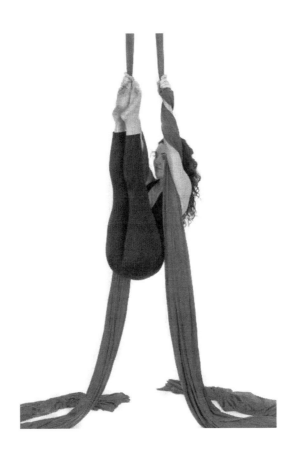

Leg Lifts

1

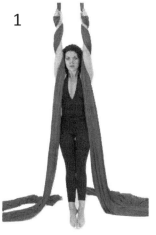

Reach your arms up high circling twice around the fabric. Hang with straight arms.

2

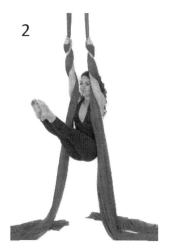

Tuck your pelvis under and begin to lift your legs.

3

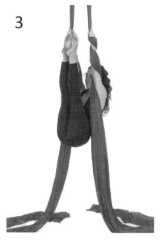

Continue to lift as high as you can maintaining straight legs and arms.

3

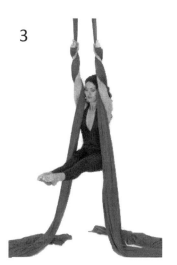

Slowly lower down.

4

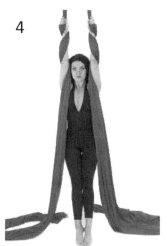

Finish with your legs under you.
Repeat 5-10x

TIPS
*Keep your legs straight the entire time! Doing so will engage the proper muscles
*Be sure not to arch your back when doing this, instead slightly tuck your pelvis under to help engage your core, hollow body position
*Hanging with straight arms will strengthen your shoulders and grip
AKA: _____

Scissors

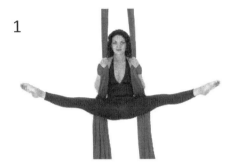

1

Choose your grip option (see pg.13). Pull up and straddle your legs to the side.

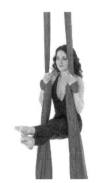

2

Scissor one leg on top of the other.

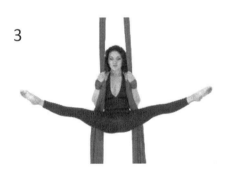

3

Open your legs into a wide straddle.

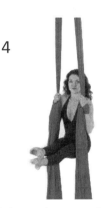

4

Scissor the opposite leg on top. Repeat 5-10x

TIPS
*Keep your elbows into your sides and your neck long
*This can be done with straight arms to strengthen your shoulders
*Work up to 10 (5 on each leg) and then add more
*It is common to feel your thighs burning after 2 reps!
* Keep your legs straight and feet pointed the entire time
AKA:_____

119

Pike Pull Ups

1

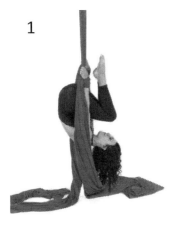

Choose your grip option (see pg. 13). Invert into a tuck.

2

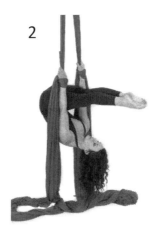

Extend your legs into a pike.

3

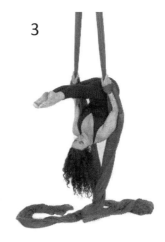

Bend your elbows as much as you can while maintaining a pike.

4

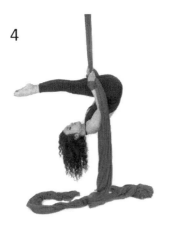

Straighten your arms. Repeat 5-10x

TIPS

*It is easy to lose your pike position when you bend your elbows, the legs may extend up, do your best not to let this happen!

*Focus on keeping your abs in, back round, leg straight and pressing together

*This is a prep for other tricks to come, it gives you the coordination and strength to do an upside down pull up

AKA:_____

Rock N Roll Tuck

1
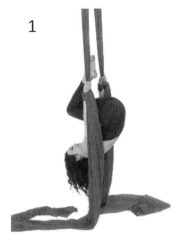

2
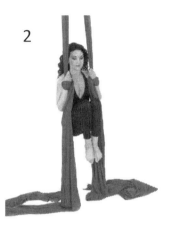

3
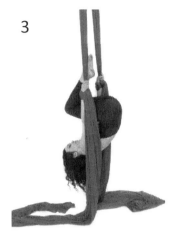

Choose your grip
option (see pg. 13).
Invert into a tuck.

Pull up, bring your
elbows into your sides
while keeping your
knees together.

Invert back into a tuck.
Repeat 5-10x

TIPS
*When pulling up bring your elbows into your sides and
pull your shoulders away from your ears to engage the
proper muscles
*Maintain a ball shape the entire time, keep your back
round and knees towards your chest
*Work up to at least 10 in a row!
AKA:_____

Rock n Roll - Single Leg

1

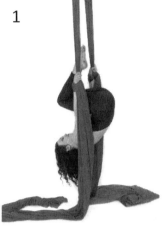

Choose your grip option (see pg. 13). Invert into a tuck.

2

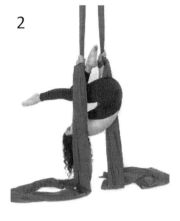

Extend one leg keeping your knees together.

3

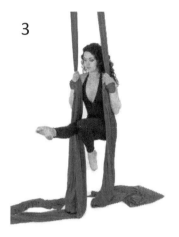

Pull up, bring your elbows in towards your sides while keeping your legs in the same shape as in step 2.

4

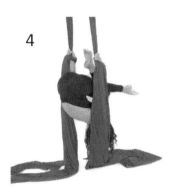

Invert back into a single leg tuck. Switch to the other leg. Repeat 5-10x on each side.

TIPS
*When pulling up bring your elbows into your sides and pull your shoulders away from your ears to engage the proper muscles
*Keep your knees together the entire time
*Work up to 10 in a row! (5 on each leg)
*Do not arch your lower back, keep your pelvis slightly tucked under to properly engage your lower abs
AKA: Seahorse

_____

Meat Hook

1

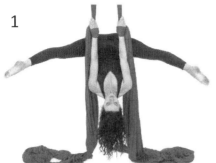

Choose your grip option (see page 13). Straddle with open fabrics.

2

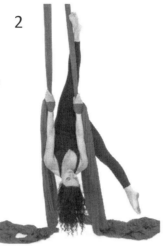

Tilt your legs to the right. Aim your right leg toward your shoulder and your left leg up on the back of the fabric.

3

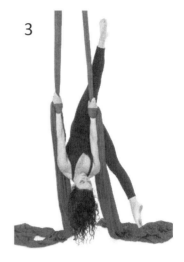

Continue to lower your left leg down to meet your right.

4

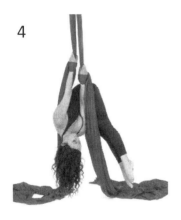

Join your legs together in a side pike position, press your top hip into your right forearm.

5

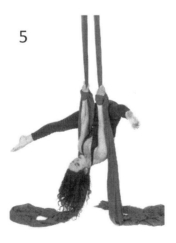

Open into a straddle.

6

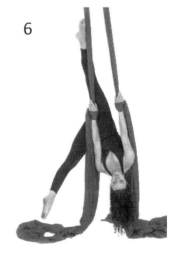

Repeat to the opposite side.

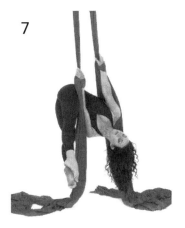

7

Join your legs together in
a side pike, press your
top hip into your left
forearm.

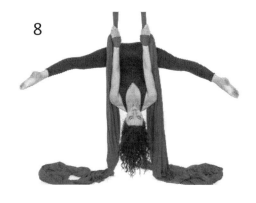

8

Return to a straddle.
Repeat 5-10x
on each side.

TIPS
*This is great for building oblique strength!
*When beginning you may find it too much to complete the full meat hook. Stop at step 2, go back to a straddle and repeat on your other side, you will still get the strength building benefits in your obliques and upper body
*Don't allow your tush to drop away from the fabric, keep your pelvis slightly tucked under and legs turned
*Be careful not to go too far with this exercise too soon, it takes a lot of strength to do with control
*Like most aerial conditioning, this exercise stems from gymnastics, the term "meat hook " literally means a *S-shaped hook or jointed hook used to hang meat*
AKA: _____

Pull Up Climb

1
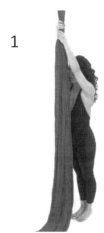

Begin standing with the fabric in front of you.

2
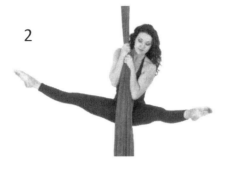

Pull up, bring your elbows toward your waist and legs into a wide straddle.

3
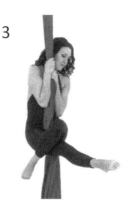

Cross one leg on top keeping the bottom leg straight and lifted.

4
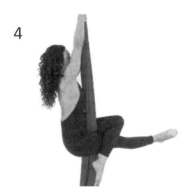

Reach your arms up high.

5
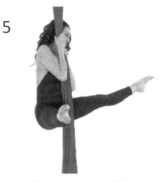

Pull up and straddle.
Repeat steps 3-4.

TIPS
*This is excellent for strengthening your upper body in preparation for no leg climbs
*Don't let your legs drop down, do your best to keep them lifted and horizontal to the floor
*Repeat with your opposite hand and leg crossed on top
*Begin with 2-3 climbs then eventually work your way to more!
AKA:_____

Pull Ups

1

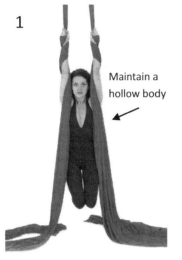

Maintain a hollow body

Choose your grip option (see page 13). Hang with straight arms.

2

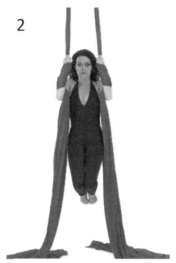

Begin to pull up.

3

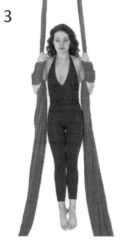

Continue to pull until your elbows are next to your waist.

4

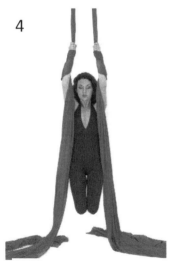

Slowly lower down.

5

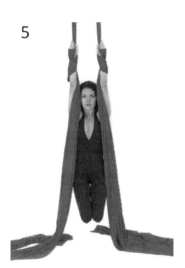

Fully hang.
Repeat 5-10x

TIPS
*Pull ups are the number one exercise to gain strength for aerial!
*Make lowering down just as important as pulling up. Work the "negative" pull up often
*Use your full range of motion to build long muscles versus short movements
*Maintain a hollow body throughout
AKA:_____

ACKNOWLEGMENTS

The author, Jill Franklin, would like to thank the following for their assistance with the production of this book:

TC Franklin Photography: www.tcfranklinphotography.com

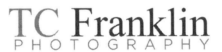

Many thanks to my aerial students and followers who inspired me to write this book. This is for you!

Lastly, a special thank you to my husband for his encouragement, support and love.

ABOUT THE AUTHOR

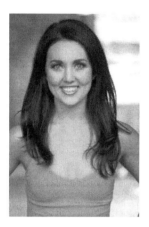

Jill Franklin, the creator of Aerial Physique is a celebrity trainer and author of *Beginners Guide to Aerial Silk* available on Amazon.com. She has a highly sought after You Tube channel, a video tutorial membership site along with a clothing line specifically for aerial work! Jill has a background in ballet, Pilates & yoga all which encompass her Aerial Physique technique. Her 5 star rated studio based in Los Angeles has attracted thousands of aspiring aerialists since 2012. Jill has over eight years of aerial experience and has been the featured aerialist for events and productions throughout the world. Jill often performs for celebrity filled galas in Los Angeles and has gracefully mesmerized audiences in productions seen on Royal Caribbean's Oasis of the Seas as well as theatres such as The Arlington Theatre-Santa Barbara, Waikiki Shell-Honolulu, Balboa Theatre-San Diego. Aerial Physique has been televised on the TODAY Show, Good Day LA, Inside Edition, Yahoo Celebrity, ABC 7 LA and many other media outlets. Jill absolutely loves helping others achieve their dream to climb and fly with ease!

BUT… It Hasn't Always Been This Way!

As a teenager I admired the aerialists in Cirque Du Soleil shows but never ever thought it was possible for me to fly through the air with such grace and ease. I assumed someone would have to begin something like that as a child. Little did I know later in life, I would prove myself wrong. At the age of 21, I moved to New York City to try my luck in the world of dancing and acting on Broadway. After a few months of pursing Broadway, I was craving something new. Aerial classes had been on my to do list for years, but I was always too scared to give it a try. I assumed it would be way too difficult for me and didn't want to look or feel silly. Finally, I decided to get over my fear and take a class. I went online, found a class, signed up and made myself go. I fell in love, instantly. In the beginning I was awful, I had no upper body strength, no sense of awareness when I was upside down, I had a huge fear of heights and the whole experience made me a nervous wreck! But there was something magical and empowering about it. So I decided to dedicate my time, effort and sweat into the art of aerial silk. In a matter of a few weeks and consistent classes, I had more strength than ever. My overall confidence in my body and in life, began to soar. Within just a couple of years, I became a professional aerialist traveling the world performing. It took patience, hard work and guts, but I achieved something I never thought possible. I hope that I can inspire you to do the same and follow your passions. Join me and introduce yourself into the exciting world of beauty, grace and strength with *Intermediate Guide to Aerial Silk.* Thank you for taking the time to read my book.

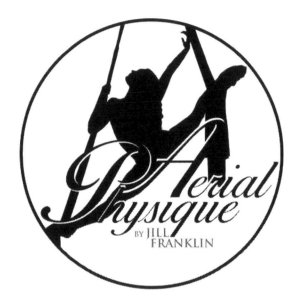

Aerial Physique offers teacher training programs, workshops worldwide as well as private and group classes at the Aerial Physique studio in Los Angeles, CA.

Visit **www.aerialphysique.com** for more information.

Contact Aerial Physique: **info@aerialphysique.com**

Keep an eye out for more books and DVDs to come!

27135114R00080

Made in the USA
Middletown, DE
12 December 2015